A GENTLER STRENGTH

A GENTLER STRENGTH
The Yoga Book for Women

Paddy O'Brien has practised and taught yoga for many years and also runs a personnel training consultancy. She runs general yoga classes and ante- and Post-Natal yoga classes. She has written many magazine articles and is the author of several books including *Birth and our Bodies* and *Your Life After Birth*. She lives in Berkshire with her partner and five children.

A GENTLER STRENGTH

The Yoga Book for Women

PADDY O'BRIEN

Illustrations by Su Eaton
Photographs by Hanya Chlala

Thorsons
An Imprint of HarperCollins*Publishers*

Thorsons
An Imprint of HarperCollins*Publishers*
77-85 Fulham Palace Road,
Hammersmith, London W6 8JB

Published by Thorsons 1991
3 5 7 9 10 8 6 4 2

© 1991 Paddy O'Brien

Paddy O'Brien asserts the moral right to
be identified as the author of this work

A CIP catalogue record for this book
is available from the British Library

ISBN 0 7225 2536 2

Typeset by Burns & Smith Limited, Derby

Printed in Great Britain by
Woolnough Bookbinding Limited
Irthlingborough, Northamptonshire

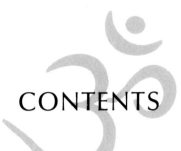

CONTENTS

DEDICATION

To S.J. O'B. with my love

ACKNOWLEDGEMENTS

My thanks are due to all the yoga teachers whose classes I have attended over the years, but especially recently to Barbara Griggs and Arjan Shahani, both of whom work constantly for understanding and exploration in yoga. I'd also like to thank all the women who have attended my classes and shared their experiences and reflections so fully.

Finally, my thanks and love to Tim.

INTRODUCTION

This book is intended as a source and introduction to yoga for women young and old, fit and unfit, beginners and experienced practitioners alike. Yoga is a huge field of deep and subtle experience and study: here I have tried simply to reflect on the aspects of yoga which feel to me to be particularly important for women.

We inhabit our beautiful women's bodies in a sexist culture in a polluted and violent world, and are often exiled both from a sense of our own beauty, and from a clear view of how to live with the dangers around us.

The pressures placed on women by our society force us to become strong in any case, but that strength is often one full of stress and tension. In the practice of yoga there is a chance to find a gentler strength with which to flow with our lives.

I first came across yoga 20 years ago completely by chance. It was the kind of chance that makes you wonder why you worry about making major decisions, because the choices which have the most radical long-term effects so often happen apparently at random: yoga changed and is still changing my life.

The impact of a teenage pregnancy had left me heavy and unfit in body and chaotic in spirit, and I had never been adept in any way at dance, gymnastics or games. However, my yoga teacher constantly emphasized the non-competitive aspect of yoga, making clear that the important part was simply to be fully present in your body, mind and spirit, at the time.

Very, very slowly, I became more supple, stronger, and lighter. At times I felt peaceful too.

Yoga has not made my life simple, or made my body a constant or ideal size and shape, or made my heart always calm. It has, however, always been with me, always been available, always been a companionable source of strength and ideas. I have done yoga in a bleak way during bleak parts of my life, and in an idyllic and joyful way when that has been the flavour of my existence.

Yoga practice has enriched my life however full or empty of grace I felt at the time I did it.

That is how it has been for me. Since everyone's experience is different I cannot tell how it will be for you. You may undergo great changes and upheavals, or startling revelations, or slow and quiet growth, or such phases may alternate. You may find in yourself qualities you never knew you had, your body may change in size or demeanour, or perhaps nothing at all will happen for some time. You do not know until you try.

I hope the ideas and suggestions in this book make a good starting place for you if you have not thought of yoga before. If you are already a student of yoga, I hope you will find material here that will interact in a new and positive way with your current thinking and practice.

chapter one

BACKGROUND TO YOGA

The word 'yoga' comes from a sanskrit word which means 'yoke' or 'something which joins or connects'. Some of the practices of yoga are known as 'hatha yoga'. 'Ha' is the sun and 'tha' is the moon, so 'hatha yoga' is 'what joins the sun and the moon'. In other words, yoga is a way of joining together and reintegrating opposites, contradictions, fragmented and broken parts of life, the yin and the yang, the warm and the cold, the swift and the slow, the sun and the moon.

Most women will recognize immediately how they have to fulfil many contradictory roles and reconcile many opposites in their lives, and see, therefore, that yoga is a wonderful resource for women. It works on many levels and you can enter into it in a cheerful open-hearted way at whatever level you feel is appropriate for you. As it becomes part of your life it will bring a deep respect and love for your own, and therefore everybody else's, body and indeed for the whole physical world, although you do not have to be uncomfortably solemn. Of course there are serious moments in the practice of yoga, but there is plenty of humour and pleasure too, so start in a light and hopeful frame of mind.

CLOTHES AND EQUIPMENT

You don't need any special equipment to begin with – all that's necessary is a clean, comfortable space and a clean blanket.

In warm weather it is pleasant to practise outside. Take care of your balance outside – indoors one unconsciously refers to the verticals and horizontals of a room in order to balance; outdoors you may feel strangely wobbly at first.

You don't need any special clothes either. You should work in bare feet both because you are less likely to slip and so that you can really feel all of your footprint on the floor. Your feet will gradually become sensitive, flexible and expressive, and you will feel the full meaning and security of the phrase 'having your feet on the ground'. Wear something which is not tight around the waist and which allows you a full range of movement and stretch in both arms and legs. If you enjoy your yoga you may want to buy a leotard or track suit or some soft trousers and tops for your practice. Instinct will guide you to choose colours which are expressive of you. In cool weather keep your practice space warm and wear plenty of layers so that you can take off layers and put them on again as you need to. Don't be misled into thinking that because you are not sweating and breathless you are not warming up and cooling down when you do your yoga: wrap up and keep warm so that your muscles can cool down slowly and gradually.

HOW MUCH TO DO, WHEN TO DO IT

Some people find it useful to practise at the same time daily or on whichever days thay choose as their 'yoga days', as they feel it keeps a steady rhythm of practice going. New students worry a great deal about how much practice to do and how they are going to 'motivate' themselves to 'keep it up', but this really is not a problem. The impulse which interests you in the first place, which prompts you to work from books and go to class, will keep you going for the first few months of your involvement with yoga. This early period is when if feels like something separate that you do a little self-consciously – 'Now I am going to do my yoga exercises'. Later on it will be the most natural thing in the world to go and do it, and you will not have to 'motivate' yourself any more than you have to motivate yourself to eat or breathe. As a rule of thumb for how long to spend on your personal practice at home, think about what is practicable within the shape of your life as it is at the moment. Anything between half an hour and two hours for a session, and anything between once and six times a week, would be sensible parameters. (Have at least one 'rest day' a week.) If you go to class and 'can't motivate yourself' to practise at home, then don't practise at home for the moment, as you obviously aren't ready to, for whatever reason. Students make tremendous progress, even when one *knows* they are not doing postures at all from one class to the next. Practising yoga *does* change you, and the impulse to *not* practise may sometimes be a hesitation in facing up to some of the changes, or a desire to slow down the rate of change. That is all right. When the time is right you will do more. This attitude of finding out from inside how much to do, rather than having it imposed from the outside, is new to most of us who have grown up in the West. However, far from leading to the floppiness and passivity which might at first seem likely, it actually generates a self-reliance and toughness. It is very important for us as women, who may well have been taught and conditioned since our time as little girls, to look for approval and validation from others. Yoga gives the responsibility to *you* to decide how long is long enough to work, how hard is hard enough to try, how well is well done. Of course one makes mistakes, sometimes painfully, but the inner strength and self-respect that come with this discipline of deciding for yourself what is your honest best on any particular day can be a wonderful antidote to a lifetime of waiting for praise or blame from parents, teachers, bosses, partners, or other powerful figures in one's life.

CHOOSING A CLASS

'When the student is ready, the teacher will appear.' There is often a striking serendipity in the ways by which people 'run into' exactly the right teacher for themselves. These ways can range from sitting next to them on the bus and, contrary to the habit of a lifetime, starting to chat to them, to walking a different way home from usual and seeing a class through a window and feeling 'drawn in'; there are all sorts of other apparent coincidences which bring together the student and the teacher who are right for one another. However, some of us have to find our teachers through the more prosaic means of contacting dance and exercise studios or yoga and fitness centres and making enquiries! When you find a class that seems to be at the right time, the right place, and the right level for you, see if you can go to just a few sessions first of all to see how you get on. Talk to the teacher about his or her background. Yoga teachers are used to being asked who their teachers were and are, what styles they have been influenced by and what their qualifications are. Mention anything special about your body, particularly any current or past back injuries or whiplash neck injuries, raised blood pressure, detached retina, or if you are pregnant. None of these conditions will prevent you from doing yoga, but there are some postures you should omit or modify, so your teacher needs to know.

The atmosphere of the class should be calm and cheerful, and there should be no sense whatever of competition or display. The teacher should be calm, competent and respectful of the students. She or he should be moving around the class at least some of the time and helping students individually – not just demonstrating at the front all the time. Apart from those guidelines, you are going to have to follow your own intuition about whether you are in the class which is right for you. There is considerable variation from class to class in the emphasis and attitude of the teacher and the style of posture practised. We all write in the same alphabet but we all have unique handwriting. The yoga postures may be the same, but everyone has a slightly different way of doing and interpreting them. You must decide for yourself whether any particular class rings true for you.

With those points in mind, do go to a class as well as working from the book if you can. Your teacher can see you in all three dimensions and from the back, which you cannot! She can therefore help you make adjustments which you would be unlikely to discover yourself. It is fun to work with other students and to learn from each other as well as sharing the ups and downs, the hilarities and frustrations which will certainly be part of the experience.

WHAT ARE THE ORIGINS OF YOGA?

Yoga is an ancient practice which originated in India. One of the oldest known pictures of someone practising a yoga pose is carved on a stone seal dating from about 2500 BC, and was found on the site of Mohenjo-Daro in the Indus Valley. Yoga was first mentioned as a technique in a collection of hymns and philosophical poetry called the *Vedas*, which were written cumulatively over a period of 2,000 years and transmitted first orally and then in a written form.

In the sixth century BC the *Bhagavadgita* was written. It is one part of a long epic poem called the *Mahabharata* and describes a dialogue between the god Krishna and the warrior Arjuna about the philosophy and practice of yoga, and it also discusses methods by which the yoga way of life can be lived.

In the second century AD the *Yoga Sutras of Patanjali* were collected and written down. *Sutra* means 'thread' (the same root word as 'suture') – the short aphorisms of the *Sutras* must be unravelled like thread to be understood, and woven together to make a whole like threads woven into a patterned fabric, in order to make a full picture. Patanjali describes yoga as an eight-fold path.

The eight paths are:

1 Laws of Life – *Yama*
2 Rules for Living – *Niyama*
3 Postures – *Asana*
4 Breathing Exercises – *Pranayama*
5 Withdrawing the Senses – *Pratayahara*
6 Concentration – *Dharana*
7 Meditation – *Dhyana*
8 Peace of Mind – *Samadhi*

These are discussed more fully in Chapters 5 and 6.

The huge time scale of the development of yoga is helpful when coming first to yoga in later years, or when one has neglected yoga for some time and is feeling stale or guilty. Yoga has been around for thousands of years. It will wait another couple of months or years for you if you need it to. It's not going to vanish overnight.

Many different styles of yoga are practised in the twentieth century. You will probably find yourself temperamentally, aesthetically, or spiritually drawn to one or other style.

A teacher who has trained in the *Iyengar* style will look very different in the postures and work in a very different way from one who is strongly influenced by the *Desikachar* approach or the *Sivananda* group's methods.

Claims and counter-claims about which is the 'best' way are not appropriate. So long as your teacher is safe, accurate and, as far as you can tell, has an authentic attitude and personal integrity, you must study the method with which you feel most 'at one'.

THE BENEFITS

Anybody who is interested in health, fitness and exercise will have spent the 1980s reading book after book about this or that system which makes stupendous claims for the method described. After exposure to all this, most of us have developed a defensive layer of cynicism. 'Oh yeah,' we think. 'Funny how *all* these techniques are supposed to be the best, the quickest, make you lose the most weight, gain the most confidence, and transform yourself the most radically.' Even more embarrassing than straight hype is hype plus obvious sniping at rival fitness programmes. In this context, how are we to describe the benefits of yoga?

Briefly, the physical benefits of yoga practice are:

- enhanced flexibility of muscles and joints
- enhanced muscular strength and power
- improved heart and lung function
- toning of immune system, glands, such as the pituitary and thyroid and of the digestive systems

The emotional benefits are:

- an ability to rebalance stresses
- an ability to get in touch with inner peace

In a way, that's all. What more could one want! There are other aspects, though, which make yoga particularly worthwhile and attractive for women. You can do yoga in all sorts of periods of your life. You can do it while you are fragile, vulnerable, undermined or exhausted, as well as when you are confident, exuberant and celebrating your strength. You don't have to be fit or supple to start with. You start from where you are at this moment.

Yoga is not a competitive form of exercise. There is terrible cultural pressure on women to be competitive in all sorts of areas, particularly weight, size and appearance. It is a great relief and pleasure to find a style of exercise that is loving and cooperative, that tunes into and enhances your own rhythms rather than imposing artificial stresses and rhythms upon you. It is a real way out of the 'rat race' of competitive living.

Although many of us begin yoga as a fitness programme, it's more than that. There is little need to say much about the compassion, peace, and inspiration yoga brings. It does it anyway, whether you speak or think consciously about it or not. By concentrating clearly, steadily and with love on your own body, insights and changes arise, sometimes obvious and spectacular, more often perhaps, subtle and diffuse. When you are making a beginning with yoga, you need not bother overmuch about these ideas. In a few months or years you will begin to look back and see what they mean to you.

If you are a long-time practitioner you will know about these positive experiences. You probably also know the long deserts and darknesses, the plateaux where nothing happens, where your body won't open or strengthen any more and your spirit sags and drifts without inspiration. We all experience those times, too. Although they make no sense at the time perhaps they are the emptiness that balance the fullness, the darkness that balances the light. Most people who have practised for a long time have had such internal struggles and despair. They may be unable to practise and unable to work out why or to talk about why for weeks or months, but they will come out of it eventually. This experience of episodes of blankness is common to all disciplines where the body is used expressively and exploratively, such as dance and the martial arts, as well as yoga. It must be in some way necessary, and it passes in time.

HOW TO USE THIS BOOK

The second chapter of this book explains and illustrates a basic series of yoga postures, which you could use as a core for your practice. The following chapters look at particular physical events and processes, and particular life events we may pass through as women, and suggest postures which may be useful at those times.

However, use the book creatively and intuitively once you have begun to feel at home with yoga. Within the guidelines of safety and balance (discussed fully in Chapter 2), you should design and evolve your own programmes.

The final chapters discuss more fully the philosophical background of yoga for women who want to reflect on and read more deeply into those aspects.

While this book is pleasant to browse through and look at, let it lead you into action too. As Swami Sivananda has said, 'an ounce of practice is worth a ton of theory': as soon as you feel you've absorbed enough to do so, begin to do some yoga for yourself, and enjoy the journey of exploration.

chapter two

PRACTICE GUIDELINES AND BASIC POSES

Here is a basic sequence of yoga poses or 'asanas' which you can use as a basis for designing your own practice.

The word 'asana' means 'seat' – and this means that it should be a comfortable position. When you first try out some of these postures you may find it amazing to think they could ever be positions of ease; however, in time, all these positions become pleasant and comfortable and the stretching sensation becomes as pleasant as an exhilarating waking-up stretch on a beautiful morning.

This sequence will take about 45 minutes at first as you will only spend a short time in each stretch. As time goes on you will find you settle for longer in each position, and this will expand the practice time to something between an hour and a quarter and an hour and a half. Even if you only have 10 or 15 minutes to spend on yoga, concentrate fully, move carefully and well, slip into your yoga frame of mind, and you will emerge refreshed as if you have had a cleansing shower after being grubby or a drink of water after feeling very thirsty.

PRACTICE GUIDELINES AND ASANAS

Move into each position slowly and carefully. Pay attention to what is going on in your body. Go to your own comfortable maximum for any particular day in each posture. Unless otherwise indicated in the description of the pose, *exhale* as you stretch into it. Remain in the pose, breathing steadily, while there is positive work happening in your body, but not so long as to feel strain or stress. Do not compete with anybody, even yourself. That is not yoga. Experience the posture fully, observe what you are feeling in it. It is through that attentive 'listening' to your body that development comes. When you are ready to move out of the posture, unless otherwise indicated, do so on a breath *in*. Come out of the pose as gracefully, slowly, and carefully as you went into it, and steady yourself for a moment or two before moving into your next stretch.

Work each side evenly – most of us begin our yoga very assymetrical: stronger on one side than the other, looser on one side than the other, more able to tell our body what to do in detail on one side than the other. If you hold a stretch for about ten seconds to the right, do about the same on the left. Gradually the two sides of the body will be increasing in equilibrium.

Do each stretch as accurately and beautifully as you can. Beautiful may not seem an appropriate word as you regard yourself struggling in the early stages of learning an asana! Remember the beauty is of genuine effort and a kind of innocence as you recover and rediscover a range of movement you undoubtedly had as a little child, but may have lost touch with as an adult. A mirror may be helpful to check yourself in face-on poses, but be careful not to twist your neck by turning to look in a mirror in a sideways-on or forward bend pose. Always think before you turn to look at any part of yourself in a pose. Would it be a natural movement for your neck to make in the position you are in? If not, ask someone else to look and tell you what is going on. A teacher will be a great help to you in describing and visualizing for you the parts of yourself you cannot see, although in some poses (e.g. *karnapidasana*, page 108) you may find yourself suddenly face to face with bits of yourself you never expected to get so close to!

Any programme you design for yourself will need a balanced sequence of asanas to give you a good stretch and expansion in all directions. All the following elements should be included in a balanced programme – a 'centred' pose (such as *tadasana* or *vrksasana*), a side stretch (such as *trikonasana* or *parsvakonasana*), a forward bend (such as *prasarita padottanasana*), a back bend (such as *bhujangasana* or *ustrasana*), a twist (such as *bharad-vajasana*), an upside-down pose (*sarvangasana*, *sirsasana*, or variations), and relaxation. Never miss the relaxation (*savasana*) at the end. If you only have 15 minutes to practise, spend 3 or 4 in relaxation. The dynamic stretching poses give us outer strength, but only *savasana* can put you in touch fully with your inner strength and resources.

BASIC SESSION

Here is a basic programme which provides a balanced cross-section of asanas.

CENTRING
Begin your session sitting cross-legged on the floor, or if *padmasana* (lotus pose) or *siddhasana* (pose of the adept) is easy for you, sit in one or other of those. Make sure you are sitting on the centre of your pelvic floor, and not sitting back on your tail bone. If you *are* sitting back on your tail bone put your hands onto your abdomen and notice that it is rather squashed in this position. Then adjust your position so that you are sitting more centrally, and see how much more space this creates in front of your body. Your inner organs are

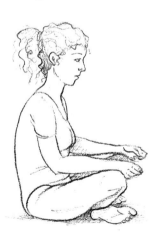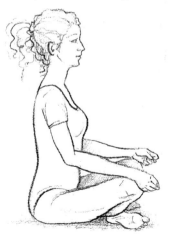

Difference between sitting centrally and sitting back on tail bone a lot happier this way and will work a lot better. If your habit is to sit back onto your tail bone it will take some weeks to gradually get back into the habit of sitting centrally and sitting tall, but you will feel a new freedom and comfort in your body as the new way of sitting becomes your natural way and not a deliberate 'exercise'.

Lift your spine, lift the crown of your head. Open your chest and release your shoulders. Feel your whole body lifting and opening. Let the backs of your hands rest on your knees. Let your eyes close.

Begin to listen to your breathing. Breathe a little more deeply and a little more slowly than usual, and hear your breath as it comes and goes. Let a slow, steady rhythm of breath develop. As you exhale, think of breathing away the distractions and tensions of the day. As you breathe in, think of drawing in with the air a feeling of serenity and calm. Exhaling, breathe away tension, inhaling, breathe in peace. Carry on in your own rhythm until you feel calm, settled, and ready to do your practice without worries and thoughts of the world flickering and darting through your mind, but with a quiet, inner equilibrium and a sense of 'calm arousal'; peaceful but alert.

The reason for sitting quietly at the beginning of your session is to ensure that you have gathered together your awareness and concentration and cleared your mind of irrelevant thoughts and mood-swings before you begin. If you remember to do this you will make fewer mistakes and very much reduce your chances of injury from jerking out of posture or making an awkward or incoherent movement because part of your mind is elsewhere. You will also have a much more satisfying time with your yoga if you are fully present with it.

When your mind is clear and settled and your body is poised, you will feel ready to 'come to' and move into the postures. Allow yourself to become aware of the place you are in, of the things around you. Let your breathing come back to an everyday level. Rub your hands together to warm them, then cover your face with your warmed hands and separate your fingers. Blink your eyes open behind your hands and let them get used to the light, before floating your hands down into your lap.

VARIATIONS
If your knees feel too stiff at first to relax in this position try sitting with one or two cushions under each knee. If there is a stiffness in

your hips, try a firm cushion, or your blanket folded up under your hips so that the back of your bottom is lifted an inch or two off the ground. If you are still too uncomfortable to sit and be calm and still your thoughts with these variations, then stretch your legs out in front of you, hip distance apart, and gently bent. Try the cross-legged position again, with cushions if necessary, in a few weeks' time. In a few weeks or months it will eventually become accessible to you.

Standing Poses

Standing poses develop strength and balance, confidence and courage. Legs become more powerful and flexible, chest and arms open and increase in mobility, and the neck strengthens and lengthens, giving poise and balance to the position of the head.

TADASANA - MOUNTAIN POSE

This is a lovely pose which grows in meaning the more you practise it. Beginning as a way of standing well, it becomes a pose in which you can sense your connection with the earth, your strength, your balance and resilience.

Bring your feet together, lining up the big toe joints. Lift your toes off the floor and wriggle them a bit before laying them back down on the floor. Send a message to your toes that you would like them to move even if nothing happens. Eventually they will move. Stand up on tiptoes for a few moments, then stretch your heels back down to the ground, having lifted the arches well.

Feel your legs strengthen and straighten as you stand tall. Feel around your pelvis to see what it is doing. If your tail bone is sticking out backwards and there is a very pronounced curve in the small of your back, try rocking your pelvis smoothly and gently forwards to tuck your tail in beneath you.

Lift your abdomen lightly up and back. As women we often have a very emotional relationship with our abdomens. Fashion dictates that we should have flat, tight boyish tummies. We dedicate ourselves to sit-ups, crunches, leg-raising, anything to eliminate any womanly roundness or softness. Ask any group of women to sit down and put their hands on their abdomens, and a look of disgust or dismay will cross many of their faces as they do it. I think it is genuinely difficult to disentangle the positive desire to have strong,

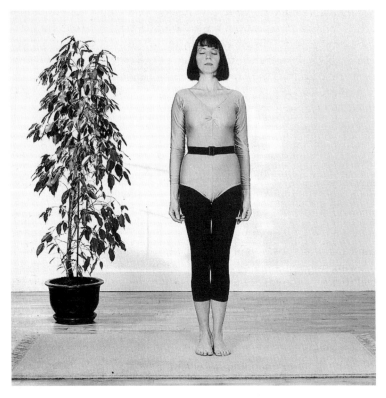

Tadasana (mountain pose)

healthy abdominal muscles and to dispense with layers of fat that feel sluggish or unpleasant, from a much more anxious desire to recreate our bodies in the image of the advertising industry's fantasy woman.

Yoga will certainly strengthen your abdomen and tighten it if it has a lot of accumulated fat which is not doing anything positive for you. However, this change is not arrived at by hating your body as it is now, or by focusing on its 'imperfections'. Therefore, for the purposes of *tadasana*, and most other postures, try not to suck your tummy in desperately or jam it angrily back towards your spine (the way one is inclined to do when catching sight unexpectedly of a round tummied profile), but try to lift it, without tension, and keep it light and active.

Lift and open your chest and release your shoulders back and down. Feel as though there is a lot of space between your ears and shoulders. Lift the crown of your head up towards the ceiling, and feel the back of your neck is long, your skull balancing on the top of your spine like a flower on a stalk.

Breathe steadily, and feel your throat is relaxed, your eyes and mouth soft, your face smooth and strong.

Now take your awareness down to your feet again. Visualize your footprints like footprints in the hard, wet sand at the edge of the sea, and try to make them even, so that you have equal weight in each foot, and equal weight between the front and the back of each foot, so you are swaying neither forwards nor backwards. Think of your feet rooting downwards through floors and ceilings, lath, plaster, concrete and foundations, down and down towards the earth. If you are outside on the grass feel your connection with the earth right away. Feel how the grass is alive, sense its roots drawing up strength. Draw up strength from the earth into yourself, feel it flow upwards through your body like sap through a plant, lifting, reviving and strengthening your body. Feel your body stretch up more lithe and alive than before. Have a real sense of yourself as a living creature, not just a walking brain or a set of symptoms or a photographic appearance. Be aware that you are made of bone and marrow, blood and sinew, muscle and gut. Sense the crown of your head is reaching, through the structure of the building if you are indoors, towards the sky, the atmosphere, the day and the night, the sun, the moon and the stars. Now you are the mountain, connecting your firm base on the earth to your peak in the sky.

Stay in the mountain pose while you feel strong and sure, and interested in what you are doing. This may not be more than ten or twenty seconds at first. Later on you may want to stay there for longer. After each standing posture, return to *tadasana*.

If you have been doing yoga for some time and always feel a bit bored in *tadasana* as though nothing much is happening, try staying there a bit longer and see if the posture begins to develop for you. If not, spend a short time there anyway in your practice, and then 'revisit' the posture for a longer time some days or weeks later. You cannot pursue meaning in yoga, all you can do is be receptive, open and aware and in time meanings emerge. You cannot 'waste time' in yoga poses, with the sole exception of poses done in a spirit of competition or anger. Any other time you spend on it will work to your benefit, in one way or another, in the end.

When you feel it is time to move out of *tadasana* step your feet a little way apart and relax (but don't collapse or slump).

TRIKONASANA - TRIANGLE POSE

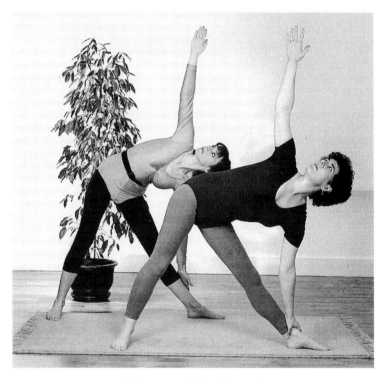

Trikonasana (triangle pose)

If you look at *trikonasana* you can see many triangles in it. The three points of the triangle represent body, mind and spirit, and the need to attend to all three.

This pose gives a lovely experience of extending the limbs and experiencing the two masses of the body – hips and shoulders – balanced with one another, together with a pleasing extension of the spine.

The particular sense of femaleness that comes during and after adolescence is a sense of two masses, the rib cage, shoulders and chest, and the wider pelvis and heavier hips which turn around a flexible waist. Relaxing into a happy sensuality has a lot to do with enjoying these two heavinesses balanced around the lightness of a mobile waist. In fact you can feel this difference in male and female bodies even in young children. When you pick up a three or four year old boy he will lift all of a piece, a kind of upward pointing arrow shape. When you pick up a little girl of the same age you can already feel the two masses of shoulders and hips and their more rounded quality.

The sculptures and drawings of Henry Moore often show these two lovely rounded shapes and their swivelling movements against each other's axes, and how beautiful they look.

Feeling and looking beautiful is much enhanced by becoming familiar with and enjoying these shapes in ourselves, and the marvellous sinuous quality of our waists. Sadly, in a culture obsessed with thinness most of us hate our waists for not being small enough, and regard our curves with anything from suspicion to deep loathing. We are aware of the lunacies of Victorian corsetry and its effect on women's health, one of its aims being to reduce radically the size of the waist, and yet few of us who lived through the 1970s did not at some time or other zip ourselves into jeans so tight that we suffered from stomach ache – goodness knows what constrictions fashion will suggest in the future. You may find that your practice of yoga does gradually alter the way you dress, particularly in terms of choosing things which do not restrict your movement.

To perform *trikonasana*, step your feet three to three and a half feet apart. Turn your left foot in about 45 degrees and your right foot out, right heel in line with left instep. Feel your feet broad and strong upon the ground and have a sense of lifting through your legs. Ensure that your bottom is not sticking out. If it is, move your tail bone forwards and down a little and give a light lift to your abdomen. Lift and open your chest, lengthen the back of your neck and let the crown of your head stretch towards the ceiling.

Inhale and stretch your arms out to the side at shoulder level. As you exhale, release your shoulders down more and stretch fully along your arms, all the way to your finger ends. Feel beautifully broad and open.

Take another breath in and stretch out to the right, extending the right side of your waist. As you breathe out, stretch to the side and down, taking your right hand to the right place for you on your right leg, going as far as you can without tilting your left hip forwards. Eventually your hand will reach the floor behind your foot. This is not the aim, it is simply the extension that will eventually come. It is far better to have your body open, supple and breathing freely, with your lower hand quite a long way up your leg, than to force your hand down to the ground, tip your hips forward, and constrict your breathing with stress.

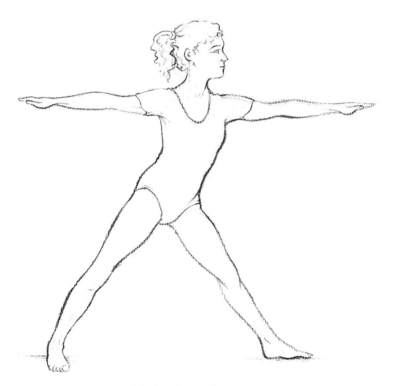

Moving into *trikonasana*

In this posture turn and look at your upper thumb with your lower eye. Breathe steadily, and keep your face and throat relaxed and your mouth soft. Be aware that the outside edge of your back foot remains firmly in contact with the floor.

When you want to come up, exhale fully, then on the breath in, come up with your arms still extended, then exhale and release your arms down to your sides.

Then turn your feet the other way and have an equally good stretch on the other side, remaining in it for roughly the same amount of time, being just as aware and observant of how it feels as on the first side.

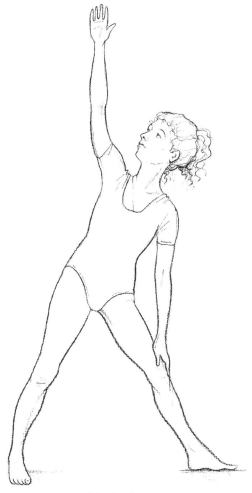

Modified *trikonasana*

PARSVAKONASANA – SIDE FLANK STRETCH
Parsva means side, and *kona* means angle. This is the extended lateral angle pose.

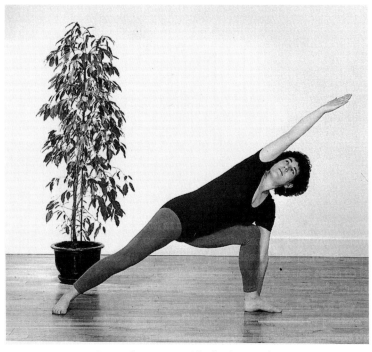

Parsvakonasana (side flank stretch)

Step your feet four to four and a half feet apart, and turn your left foot in about 45 degrees and your right foot out, with your right heel in line with your left instep. Feel your feet in firm contact with the floor, and bring a strong sense of lifting and life up through your whole body.

Prepare to go into the pose by resting the back of your right hand against your right knee to encourage your hips to stay open. Bend your right knee, trying to make a right angle between thigh and calf – thigh parallel to the floor and shin vertical. Take care not to extend your knee beyond your front foot. Having checked that your stance is the right width and felt out the correct position for your bent leg, come up again to begin the pose.

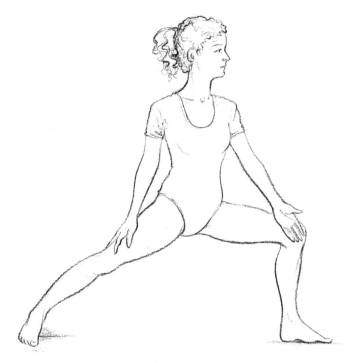

Preparation for *parsvakonasana*

Inhale, bringing your arms out to the sides at shoulder level, and exhale, stretching down to the finger tips, shoulders releasing down. Feel your body is alive all through. Be aware of your back and neck being straight and long, your abdomen lifting, your legs strong. On your exhalation, bend your right knee into the position you have practised, extend the lower side of your waist, and move your hand either into the position on the floor, as in the photograph, or bend your right elbow and rest it on your knee as in the drawing. As you breathe in stretch your left arm up, and over your head. Press the outside of your back foot into the floor, and feel your back and waist stretch. Experience the wonderful stretch from the outside of your left foot right through to your left fingertips, and try to keep your lower waist stretching too (it may tend to collapse a little at first). Turn and look up from under your upper arm. Breathe steadily and keep your face and throat soft, your neck long.

When you feel it is the right time for you to come out of the pose, exhale fully, and then inhale and come up. Exhale and lower your arms to your sides. This is a strong pose, and five or ten seconds will be plenty to remain in it at first. Later on you may want to stay for half a minute or a little longer.

Do *parsvakonasana* to the other side, for about the same length of time, and be sure to experience it just as fully on the second side.

You will feel longer in the waist, stronger in the legs, and freer in the chest and arms after practising *parsvakonasana*.

VIRABHADRASANA II – WARRIOR POSE II

Virabhadra is one of the warrior poses, Virabhadra being the name of a fierce and brave warrior.

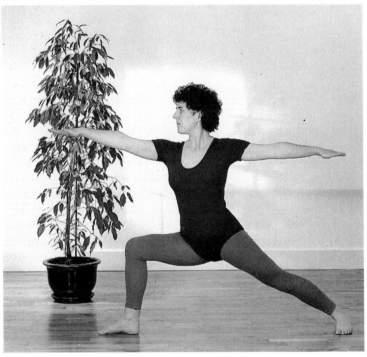

Virabhadrasana II (warrior pose II)

Prepare and check your stance for this posture in the same way as you did for *parsvakonasana*. When your stance feels right, and you know that when you bend the front knee you will have your shin vertical and your knee above, but not beyond your foot, you are ready to begin.

Inhale and stretch your arms out to the side. As you breathe out, release your shoulders and extend, stretching broad and strong out into your fingertips, and at the same time bend your front knee, with the shin vertical and the thigh working towards being parallel to the floor. Keep strong in your back leg and ensure that the outside edge of your back foot remains in contact with the floor. Keep your left hip open and your chest open and strong. Look to the right.

A common problem with this pose is to have the line from fingertip to fingertip tilting either to the back or the front. Check in a mirror or ask someone to align your arms. When you feel you want to come out of the stretch, inhale and come up, and exhale, floating your arms down to your sides. Afterwards practise with equal attention and strength on the other side.

This pose is strong and vigorous. Imagine yourself as you do it being the warrior Virabhadra. You are astride a magnificent war horse. In the distance is the noise and tumult of battle. You are about to join the battle to fight for what you passionately believe is a righteous cause. As you exhale and bend the front knee imagine you have gathered your courage together and set off at a gallop into the fray. You will find this visualization sends a shiver of courage through your body and enables you to do a strong and brave stretch.

Your legs are strengthened, and your arms, chest and hips have an open feeling. Also, even the most timid of us begins to get in touch with the warrior within as we practise the warrior poses. Few women get through their lives without needing to fight many battles, though they may not be obvious or physical ones. While you practise warrior stretches allow yourself to be aware of the courage you have had in your own battles and the strength needed to get through even an apparently ordinary and uneventful life. It is useful sometimes to stop, appreciate and celebrate this strength, and also to begin to observe these kinds of courage in the other women in our lives.

VRKSASANA – TREE POSE

Vrksasana is a balance executed on one leg, and its name means the pose of the tree. If you feel insecure while learning to balance, place one hand against the wall to help you. In time you will be able to balance without support.

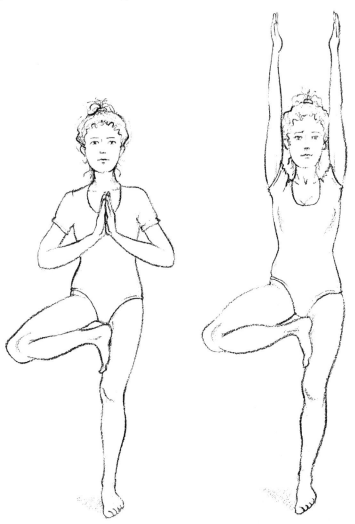

Vrksasana (tree pose) in *namaste*   *Vrksasana* with arms overhead

Start in *tadasana*. Step forwards a few inches with your right foot. As you put the foot down, notice the contact with the floor by pressing into your heel and then spreading your toes out before putting them down. Think of roots spreading down into the ground.

Now bend your left knee and place your left foot on the right place for you on your right leg. If you feel very shaky you can begin by placing your foot over your ankle or knee. Eventually you will be able to place your left heel right up into the opposite groin. Place the back of your left hand on the front of your left bent knee for a few moments to encourage your left hip to open more fully and your knee to move backwards so that it is, eventually, in the same plane as your pelvis.

Be aware of smoothly tucking in your tail bone and lifting your abdomen. Feel your chest is open and your shoulders relaxed. Lift

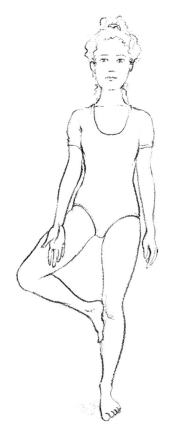

Modified *vrksasana*

through your spine from where it rises out of the pelvis right up to the base of your skull.

Steady your gaze on an object straight ahead. A spot or mark on the wall will do, but if you are practising at home you may like to find something beautiful to look at – flowers, a stone, a shell, or a crystal. Steadying your gaze will help you to steady your balance.

When you feel balanced, put your hands together in *namaste* (placing your hands in the prayer position in front of your heart). Imagine the tree that you become in the pose, rooted well into the ground, and life and nourishment flowing up from the roots to the tip of the highest leaf. If you feel safely balanced, inhale and stretch your arms out to the sides, then exhale and stretch them straight up, palms facing each other, taking care not to let your shoulders hunch up close to your ears. Keep your gaze steady and your breathing soft. Do not tighten your jaw!

Notice the qualities of a tree – flexibility and strength. Notice how the pose will enhance those qualities in your body, and hence in your life. Also, observe which kind of tree came into your mind when you began to visualize a tree. Did you think of a rugged pine, a graceful silver birch, a solid oak, a weeping willow, a horse chestnut laden with flowers – or some other of the many species? Think of which one came spontaneously into your mind, and see what message it has for you, what particular qualities it has. They will be particularly relevant to you in some way at this moment, and it may be useful to you to reflect on what that is.

When you wish to come out of the pose, exhale and stretch your arms out and down to your sides. Carefully disengage your left foot. You may like to hug your right knee up towards you for a few seconds if there is any tension in it. Now stretch into *vrksasana* standing on your left foot, being careful to stretch, lift and elongate as fully as before, and to open your hip as fully as possible on the right.

Return to *tadasana*.

PRASARITA PADOTTANASANA – WIDE STRIDE STRETCH

In this powerful stretch the feet are spread wide apart, the legs well stretched, the spine lengthened and extended, and the hips rotated strongly. It is a positive, expansive, and energizing posture.

Begin in *tadasana*, then step your feet in a wide stride, four to four and a half feet apart. Feel your broad, strong feet in full contact with the floor.

Place your hands on your hips and stretch up strongly through your whole spine, lift your abdomen lightly and firmly. Your shoulders stay relaxed and your chest open.

Inhale and grow still a little taller, pressing your foot down, and stretching the crown up. Exhale and stretch forwards with a broad, flat back, hinging at the top of your legs (never in any forward bend, from the back of your waist). Continue to extend forwards until you cannot go forwards any more (keeping your hips above your feet), and then begin to release down, keeping your back and the back of your neck long. Place your hands on the floor.

Keep a firm footing and a feeling of lifting up through the backs of your legs. Do not let the front of your body feel bundled up – let it stay free and open.

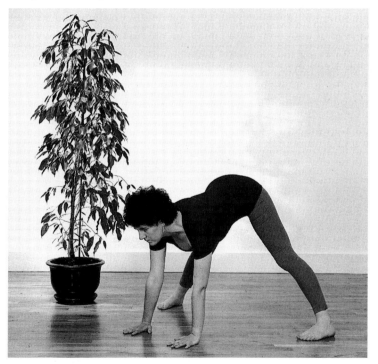

Prasarita padottanasana (wide stride stretch)

Eventually your head and elbows will rest comfortably on the floor.

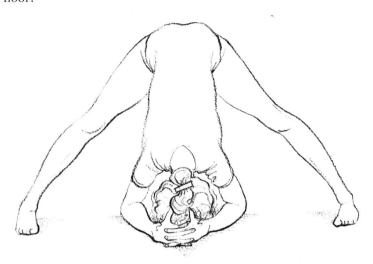

Advanced *prasarita padottanasana*

If, at first, your hands do not reach the floor, hold on to opposite elbows and let the weight of your arms ease you further down.

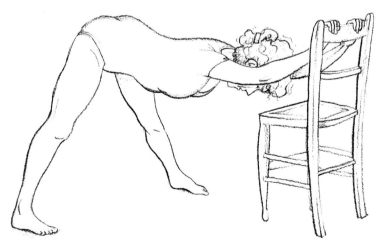

Modified *prasarita padottanasana*

When you want to come out of the posture, wriggle your feet in a few inches. Breathing in, lift your head and exhaling, press your abdomen back towards your spine, and come up.

VARIATION
If you have a lower back injury do not stretch all the way down in this pose. Simply go forwards until your torso is parallel to the floor, and rest your hands with arms extended, or folded arms, on a heavy piece of furniture (a work top or heavy table which will not slip). Concentrate on spreading your back broad and flat, and strengthening your abdominal muscles by flexing them back towards your spine. Feel your legs strong, stretched, and lifting. When you want to come out of your stretch, inhale and lift your head, then exhaling, *walk towards the support* so you do not stress your back when coming up.

Back bends

These two back bends open and stretch the front of your body, and also flex the spine in a backwards stretch. Be careful and observant of your body in these postures and do not go any faster than your body wants to go. Do not get discouraged if you feel stiff and immobile, as little by little the impossible happens, and where you started off feeling like a block of concrete, you will eventually feel light, springy, and flexible.

You should read carefully the following advice before starting practice on any back bends.

- Do not do powerful back bending postures in the second and third trimesters of pregnancy unless you are already very experienced in yoga.
- If you have recently experienced back strain or injury, move very slowly and attentively into a gentler version of any back bending posture, and avoid holding your breath.
- Be sure to do the counter posture, praying stretch (page 41) and release your back fully.
- An astounding eighty per cent of adults in the affluent West have back problems of one kind or another. Careful practice of forward and back bends (it is important to do both) is protective of the health of your spine.

BHUJANGASANA - COBRA POSE

Bhujanga is a serpent. *Bhujangasana* is often called the cobra pose, as the upper body eventually lifts off the ground like a cobra preparing to strike.

Lie down on the floor face downwards with your knees and feet together. Place your palms on the floor on either side of your chest, with your fingers pointing forwards.

Inhaling, lift your face from the floor, and exhaling rise up off the floor like a snake, keeping your pubic bone on the floor, and being aware of your tail bone moving in and down. Use back and body strength to lift your body up – do not push into your hands, think of them as simply an aid to your balance. You will feel a lot of work in your hips and thighs, and maybe in your arms too. Look straight ahead and think of being quick and sinuous like a snake. Be careful to keep your shoulders relaxed. It is better to have bent elbows and relaxed shoulders and an open chest, than to have straight arms and a tense chest and collar bone.

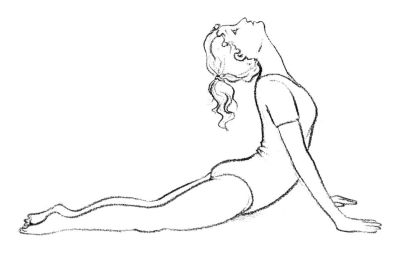

Bhujangasana (cobra pose)

Perhaps at first you will only lift off the floor a couple of inches, or perhaps you will feel what seems a ridiculous weakness in your forearms, especially if your weight is falling forwards into your hands. If so, only stay in the stretch for a couple of breaths, and do not despair. It may take months, it may take a couple of years, but unlikely though it seems just now, you will eventually open up like a flower!

When you have had enough stretch in this pose, flow forwards and down back onto the floor, and rest your face to one side, and your arms along your sides. Let your breathing and your heartbeat come back to normal.

When you have had a short rest, repeat the pose, and when you lie down again, rest your face on the alternate side. After your breathing and heart rate have settled again, push up onto all fours, then sit back on your heels and rest in the praying stretch.

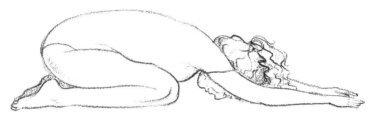

Praying stretch

This will remove any tension in the back of your waist and your lower back. In the praying pose, spread out in the lower back, and keep the front of your body as long as possible as well as stretching along your spine. Keep the back of your neck long. It may take some time before your body folds comfortably over itself in the praying pose, but again, don't feel disheartened, regular stretching will soon ease it out.

If you are far too stiff to fold forwards along your thighs at the moment, then sit back onto your heels, and fold your arms onto the seat of a chair, resting your head down onto your arms, gradually increasing the flexibility in your spine.

USTRASANA - CAMEL POSE
This is a more intense back bend: its name means the pose of the camel.

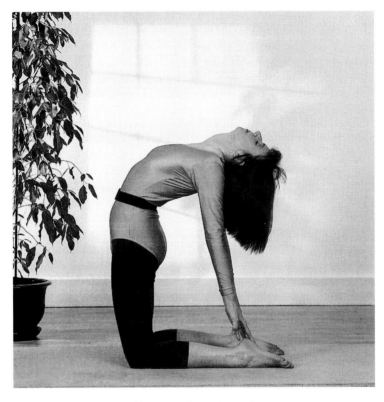

Ustrasana (camel pose)

Kneel on the floor. At first you may find the pose easier with your knees a few inches apart, and your toes curled under and pressing into the floor. As you find more stretch, try to do it with your knees together and the tops of your insteps on the floor.

Inhaling, stretch your spine upwards, lengthening up out of your hips until your thighs are vertical. Tuck in your chin and place your hands flat on the back of your hips. Stay in this position, keeping your chin on your chest and begin to lean your upper body backwards, thinking of eventually having your torso parallel to the floor. Gently lower your arms until your fingers touch your heels. When it feels safe and appropriate, slowly let your head fall back, keeping the neck long.

You may not go backwards very far at first, and you may find it useful to have a chair behind you.

Eventually your spine will stretch enough for you to reach back and hold your heels. Keep pushing your hips forwards, and, lengthening your neck, let your head stretch back. Think of the front of your body opening out like a spinnaker sail.

Breathe steadily. As always, maintain a softness in your face and neck. It is easy to begin to clench your teeth when you are concentrating hard: try not to let this happen, but if it does, exhale and soften your jaw. The habit of coping with intense effort and concentration, or intense sensation, with calm breathing and a calm expression, will soon spill into the rest of your life, and you will find yourself wasting much less energy by uselessly clenching fists, facial muscles, or feet and legs, when you are in conflict or under pressure.

There are two ways out of the camel pose. When you feel confident and strong, come up on an inhalation, taking your thoughts to your abdominal muscles so that their strength lifts you up, rather than your back muscles. After getting to an upright kneeling position, sit smoothly back down onto your heels, then stretch forwards into the praying stretch, as you did after *bhujangasana*.

If coming up that way feels risky, exhale and lift your head and chest up as you slowly sit your bottom back down onto your heels. Lengthen forwards into the praying stretch as before.

After a short rest, do the posture again.

These back bends are stimulating for your spine, and also make the front of your body feel fresh and alive.

Another quality of back bending postures is that they help to recover movements and positions which we all enjoyed as children, and tend to lose as adults. Back bending and arching seldom appear in other sports and disciplines, and are rarely, if ever, postures we need to get into for everyday tasks and chores.

The cobra pose is one of the first positions little babies get into in their carrycots as they press their hands and arms down and rear their heads up to peer at the world around. Older children exult in back arching and are often able to walk or scuttle around in the 'crab' position (yoga pose *urdhva dhanurasana*) just for fun, or walk their hands backwards down the wall behind them, ending up in an arched position. Perhaps it is the exultation we feel in these positions as young children that gives them such a carefree feel.

Sitting poses

Sitting poses bring a lightness and flexibility to the hips and legs, and many of them give a composed and comfortable position for the body to rest in while you practise meditation or *pranayama*. Many of them can simply become ordinary ways of sitting when you sit on the floor: and sitting on the floor more frequently will increase your flexibility and mobility anyhow.

DANDASANA - STAFF POSE

Sit on the floor with your legs extended straight out in front of you, heels pushing away. Pull your hips back to make sure you are sitting on the centre of your pelvic floor, then lift up through the whole of your spine, also lifting your abdomen and relaxing your shoulders. Lift the crown of your head and keep your chin in so that your neck is long.

Place the palms of your hands on the floor at hip level, fingers pointing forwards, and begin to straighten your arms, although it is better to have your shoulders relaxed and your elbows slightly bent, then to have your arms straight and your shoulders hunched.

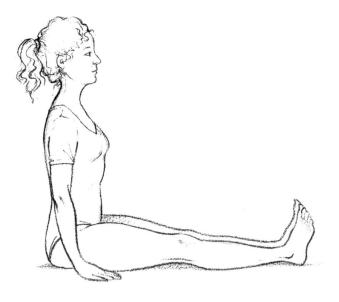

Dandasana (staff pose)

Dandasana means 'staff pose' and your spine should lift up as straight as a staff or stick. In drawings or photographs it may look as though nothing much is happening in this pose, but when you try it, you find that there is a great deal of activity. The tops of your thighs may quiver and protest, while the back of your waist may have an irresistible desire to curve back towards the floor, so that the front of your abdomen is squashed and collapsed. Little by little these discomforts pass and you can sit freely in *dandasana* as a strong upright posture. When you've had enough, come out of the pose by relaxing, but not collapsing.

Dandasana inculcates in the body a habit of sitting tall with the spine stretched up and the abdomen lifting and free, so that the circulation and workings of the soft inner organs are improved. What starts as an enormous effort gradually becomes a natural way to sit in any circumstances, not just while 'doing yoga', which brings health to your whole body.

If *dandasana* is so uncomfortable that it is impossible to hold it at all, fold your blanket into a firm rectangular block and sit on the edge of it, lifting your bottom a few inches off the ground. As it gets easier, gradually have fewer and fewer folds of blanket under you, until you are ready to sit on the floor.

PASCHIMOTTANASANA – STRONG FORWARD STRETCH

Begin in *dandasana* for this deep forward bend. Breathe in and sit up tall, out of your hips. Slide your hands down the outsides of your legs to wherever you can hold on comfortably without beginning to round your shoulders. Keep your head up. At your comfortable maximum, release your head and neck. Make sure the movement of your spine is forwards, not rounding downwards. Your chin will eventually rest on your shins, rather than your forehead going down onto your knees. Don't be tempted to bounce to get down further; on the breaths out simply relax further into the stretch, emphasizing the extension *forwards*. If it is very difficult to make any forward movement you could loop a scarf round your feet and pull steadily on it to help yourself loosen up. Be careful not to round down and constrict your abdomen. To come up, breathe in and lift your head, then exhale and come up with your back flat and broad.

At first this is a most frustrating posture. I remember clearly feeling furious at my hip joints which refused to make anything but

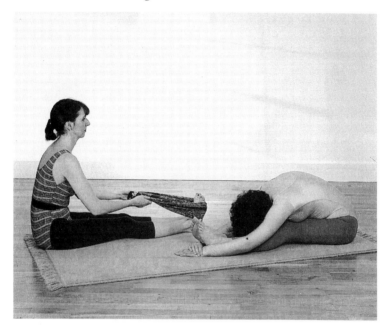

Paschimottanasana (strong forward stretch) and modified
paschimottanasana with scarf

the most marginal swivelling movement forwards, and listening to
my teacher saying 'feel a stretch but not a strain', wondering which
of those the excruciating pain up the backs of my legs was supposed
to be. Now I find this pose positively pleasurable and relaxing, and
where at first my heart sank when it was time to do it, these days I
look forward to it.

Yogis used to practise facing the rising sun, so the front of the
body is known as the East, and the back of the body is known as the
West or *Paschima*. The whole of the back of your body, from heels
to head, is stretched in the pose. The abdominal muscles are toned
and massaged in this posture too.

UPAVISTHA KONASANA – WIDE ANGLE STRETCH
Begin in *dandasana*. Stretch your legs as wide apart as you can. Find
the optimum point where you are extending your legs apart but have
not fallen back onto your tail bone – make sure you are still sitting
well into the centre of your pelvic floor, and lifting out of your hips.

Open your chest, release your shoulders, and keep your neck long, head lifting up from the crown. Rest the backs of your hands on the fronts of your knees. Breathe steadily, move your hands to the floor between your legs. Try to forward bend from this position – inhaling, make the back and the front of the body long and open, then exhaling, stretch forwards and down, walking your hands out in front of you. Remember to hinge at the hips and not the waist, and not to feel too depressed if at first you go no more than a couple of inches forwards. Little by little the impossible *will* happen.

BADDHA KONASANA – COBBLER POSE (ILLUSTRATED ON PAGE 74)

Sitting tall, bring the soles of your feet together and bring them as close to the perineum as you can. Interlink your fingers and cup them round underneath your feet. Release your knees down towards the floor, again being careful not to fall back onto your tail bone as you stretch your thighs further apart. Lift your spine and keep your chest open, and lift from the crown of your head.

This pose gives a lovely feeling of stretching and opening in the hips. Circulation is stimulated in the pelvis. At first it is difficult to keep your spine free and lifting in *baddha konasana*; it tends to curve back, but after a while you can arrive at a strong upward movement and sense of expansion in your chest as well as a serene expression.

VIRASANA – HERO POSE

Virasana gives a pleasing counter-movement to the wide abduction of the thighs in *upavistha* and *baddha konasana*. Many women enjoy sitting in this position naturally anyway, and are surprised to find that it is a yoga pose!

Kneel up with your knees together and separate your feet wide enough for your hips to fit between them. Slowly sit down between your feet. If, half-way down, your knees begin to protest and feel very tight, then kneel slowly up again. Arrange a couple of cushions, or your blanket folded into a firm rectangular lift, between your feet, and try again. You will find it is much easier if you do not have to go down so far. Gradually decrease the height of your 'lift' as your knees and upper thighs become more flexible. Sometimes the tops of the insteps are extremely uncomfortable at first: a flannel or soft cloth between the foot and the floor may help, and again, time will ease your feet into a more flexible state as you continue to practise.

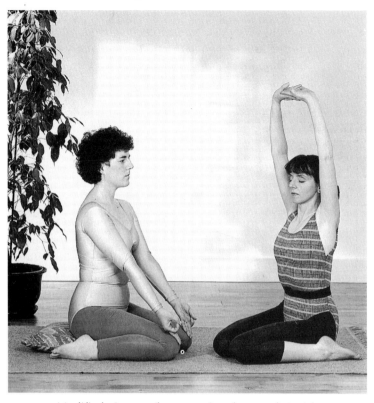

Modified *virasana* (hero pose) and upward stretch

When you have your hips and legs settled, sit up tall. Link your fingers together, exhale, and stretch your arms out and up, over your head if possible, but be careful to be aware of the flexibility of your shoulders, and only go to the right place for you. Think of releasing your shoulders down away from your ears, and keep your face smooth and relaxed, your mouth and throat soft. Stay in the posture, breathing steadily, until you want to come down. Exhale, and float your arms slowly down into your lap. Look at your hands: you will have automatically linked them with one index finger on the top. Change, and link your hands again with the other index finger on top (it will probably feel very odd!). Have another slow stretch up.

Virasana is the pose of the hero. Any time we read of women's lives in the past, or have a chance to hear about women's lives now from each other and from the media, we are struck by their heroism. This posture is a good chance to remember and celebrate any strong, heroic women by whom we have been inspired, and also to acknowledge the heroism in our own lives.

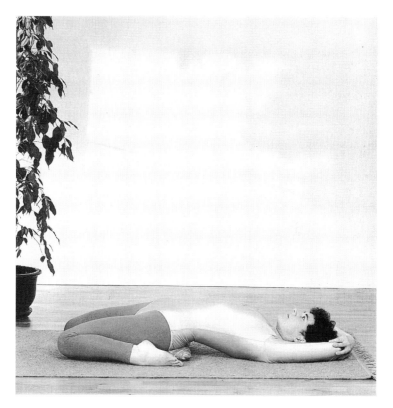

Modified *virasana supta*

After the upward stretch, try lying back in *virasana supta*. Until your knees, thighs and spine are accustomed to this stretch, arrange two or three large pillows or cushions behind you, and rest back onto these. Hold onto your feet, and exhaling, sink back onto one elbow, then the other, then unwind your shoulders and head onto the pillows. When you are ready to, you can uncurl down onto the floor in full *virasana supta*, then let go of your feet and stretch your arms up over your head. A wonderful feeling of lengthening comes into the front of your body.

You can come up by reversing the steps by which you got down, or by lifting first one foot, then the other, placing them on the floor with your knees bent, and finally rolling over onto your side and pressing your hands into the floor to lift yourself up.

BHARADVAJASANA II - TWISTING POSE

Bharadvajasana II is one of the twisting postures. Start in *dandasana*.

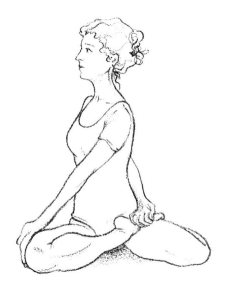

Bharadvajasana II (twisting pose)

Bring your left heel in towards your perineum. If you can comfortably do so, lift it onto your right thigh in half lotus position. Bend your right knee and tuck your right foot round behind you next to your hip, as in *virasana*, the hero pose.

When twisting, work from the base up. Think of the twist travelling up your spine like a person walking up a spiral staircase. Exhaling, begin to twist to your left, spiralling up from the root of your spine up to the top of your head. Take the back of your right hand to the left of your left knee. Slide your left hand round behind your waist – eventually you will be able to hold the toes of your left foot (the one in half lotus) as you twist around. Breathe steadily and think of keeping your brow smooth and your mouth and throat soft. Keep the back of your neck long and graceful. After you have stayed as long as feels right, exhale and release, slowly uncoiling back to the centre. Repeat the twist in the other direction, remaining in the twist for about the same length of time.

This twisting action increases mobility in the spine, and squeezes and massages the abdominal organs. The mobility and flexibility in the waist gives a confidence and resilience to your style of movement and behaviour.

Salamba Sarvangasana – SHOULDER STAND

As a child you may have spent many happy times upside down – hanging from climbing frames, doing handstands, standing on your head. Many of us spent the last few weeks before being born resting in a head-down position! The inverted postures give us a chance to get used to being upside down once again.

Don't do upside down postures during a menstrual period (there is a theoretical possibility of the flow, being reversed, trickling back into the abdominal cavity). See page 74 for discussion of inverted postures during pregnancy. If you have not spent much time upside down since your childhood, approach the pose in easy stages, as in these illustrations.

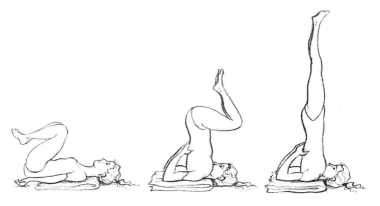

Step-by-step *salamba sarvangasana* (shoulder stand)

Once you are in a comfortable balance in shoulder stand, refine the pose by lifting more and more up through your spine and making your legs stretch up vertically above your hips. Your elbows should stay no more than shoulder distance apart. Push your heels towards the ceiling, to elongate fully along the backs of your legs, and then relax your feet so that your toes are uppermost.

There are many benefits to be gained from practising *salamba sarvangasana*: the thyroid and parathyroid glands are massaged because the chin is pressed into the base of the throat, and function healthily, constipation and headaches are relieved, and the upside-down position refreshes the legs by taking pressure off the valves in the veins – in fact *sarvanga* means 'the entire body' and this is a posture that benefits all parts.

Twenty or thirty seconds may be plenty for this position at first – gradually increase the time you spend there. To come down, bend your knees, then uncurl onto the ground vertebra by vertebra, supporting yourself with your hands as you go.

When your back is on the floor place first one foot flat on the floor with your knee bent, then the other. Slide first one leg, then the other, slowly out straight. Think of your lower back spreading out. If you do feel a tightness there, slowly hug your knees back onto your chest again, and rock gently from side to side until any discomfort is gone.

Awareness of Breathing

From birth till death we breathe, steadily and continuously – sleeping, waking, dreaming, still or moving. It is one of our ways of interacting and exchanging materials with the universe in which we live. Except at times of severe illness or emergency, this interaction takes place spontaneously and without any conscious effort on our part.

When we begin to do yoga postures we become aware of our breathing. We generally exhale as we stretch, inhale as we come up out of a stretch, and learn to breathe steadily and evenly even when in an intense stretch. Gradually the habit of exhalation on an effort, and continuing to breathe in a slow and steady rhythm even while under stress, spreads out into other parts of our lives. We learn to react to conflict or challenge not by a sharp intake of breath and clenched muscles, but with easy breathing and a strong, loose physical stance. Try these awareness exercises to extend your consciousness of your own breathing. There is a branch of yoga known as *pranayama*, connected with breathing awareness, but these awareness exercises are not really *pranayama* – *pranayama* is fundamentally to do with developing an awareness and control of *prana*, or life-energy, addressed through the movement and action of the breath.

ABDOMINAL BREATHING

This exercise helps to remind your body of the way you breathed deeply and easily as a little child – when your whole lungs filled and moved your diaphragm down so that your tummy expanded out when you breathed in, and deflated a little when you breathed out. Anxious adults often breathe only in the upper branches of their lungs, so that their abdomens suck in while they breathe in and their chests puff out; then as they breathe out, their abdomens sag forwards and their chests sink. See what your present pattern of breathing is, and whether this feels different.

Sit with your legs comfortably crossed, or supported as in 'centring' (page 21). If you are really comfortable in half lotus, lotus, or *siddhasana*, you could sit in one of these positions. Lift up tall out of your hips, and feel the back of your neck is long. Let your shoulders release back and down. Place both hands on your lower abdomen. Let your eyes close.

Begin to give attention to your breathing. Don't do anything to it, just listen, watch, be aware. Once your rhythm is settled and steady, slow it down a little, but not so much that it becomes a strain.

After a while, become aware of your hands on your tummy. Imagine that you are sending the breaths in down towards your hands, so that your abdomen swells into your hands a little. When you breathe out, imagine the breath comes from behind your hands, and let your abdomen collapse back a little. When you breathe in, you fill up, so your abdomen swells a little. When you breathe out you empty, so your abdomen falls back a little.

Take your awareness round your body, and notice whether you have tensed up the back of your neck, your shoulders, or your calves and thighs, or tightened up hands, arms or waist, because you are concentrating on how to breathe. If a tightness has appeared somewhere, notice it, and on an exhalation, let it go. Be soft around your mouth and eyes.

Be aware if your tummy is rising and falling the opposite way round from usual (i.e. if you usually suck it in on a breath in, and let it go on a breath out). If so, this way will feel strange at first, but will gradually become your 'usual' way, and will make a fuller kind of breathing an ordinary part of your life.

As you settle into your abdominal breathing, feel how still your body and mind become.

Try to inhale and exhale at a steady rate – imagine you are filling a container with liquid at an even rate, and pouring it out again, equally evenly. See if you can make the inhalation and the exhalation last an equal amount of time. Think of the air flowing in, the exchange of gases in your lungs, the new oxygen taken into your bloodstream, the gases you don't need flowing out. Be aware of the perspective this gives you about one aspect of your presence in the world. Think of the forests absorbing sunlight and breathing out oxygen into the atmosphere.

When you feel ready to stop, gently take your hands away from your abdomen and rest them on your knees. Let your breathing come back to an everyday level. Become aware of your present surroundings. Only when it feels right for you, blink your eyes open and gradually let in the light. Do not jump up and rush around. Have another few minutes of quietness before you return to the activities of your day.

If you ever become dizzy doing this or any other breathing exercise, return at once to an everyday level of breathing. If you try the same exercise again at a different time, do not 'try' quite so hard or breathe so vigorously. It is as harmful and inappropriate to force your breathing as it is to force your joints and muscles in physical stretching.

REVITALIZING BREATHING

This coordinated breathing and stretching exercise is a good way to revive flagging energies if you are feeling sluggish or low.

Begin by sitting on your heels, then lifting your spine and abdomen and lengthening the back of your neck. Spread out across your upper chest and release your shoulders. Exhale.

On your breath in, kneel up, stretch up your arms, and stretch right through to the ends of your fingertips. Make the breath last the same amount of time as the stretch, so that the breath and the stretch

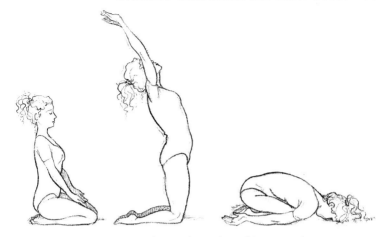

Three stages of revitalising breathing exercise

are one. Exhale with a 'whooshing' noise through your mouth and stretch forwards and down. As you lie along the tops of your thighs take your arms back alongside your body. This is known as the pose of the child, an informal resting posture. Again, make the movement and the breath last the same amount of time, and a matching degree of intensity, so that the movement and the breath are united.

After half a dozen cycles or so, sit back on your heels again, sitting tall and graceful, and feel the new energy in your body and mind. Allow your breathing to return to an everyday level, and collect your thoughts before moving on to the tasks of your day.

The same cautions about dizziness and forcing the breath apply as those mentioned in 'abdominal breathing'. Work in every kind of yoga with a calm, alert observance, and you will not hurt yourself.

MEDITATION

Do not fear that meditation is an esoteric activity which you will probably not be able to do, or will certainly not be able to do properly. Meditation is not a strange activity, it is something we have all done spontaneously anyway, and the point of sometimes choosing to do it deliberately is, again, to make this calming, healing and strengthening activity more of a part of our lives.

During most of our waking hours our minds rattle around

restlessly from one subject to another, one enthusiasm to another, one anxiety to another. Any time we become absorbed in an activity so that our mind is focused upon that one thing, we are freed from the kaleidoscope of outside distractions. We feel happy and peaceful at the time, and refreshed and revived afterwards. At other times we slip into a kind of spontaneous trance. You may gaze out of the train or bus window, and find with surprise that hours of the journey have passed while your mind has been in some other sphere. You may have sat gazing into the distance with your hands resting on your pregnant belly, feeling kicking and flickering baby movements under your hands, your thoughts 'miles away', or done familiar and mechanical work while your thoughts are free to clear, and float in unharassed free space. These are all examples of spontaneous meditative practices.

EXERCISE IN MEDITATION

To practise meditation, begin by finding a comfortable sitting position – either crosslegged, or in half-lotus (page 57) or lotus (page 67) if you are really comfortable in either of those. Rest the backs of your hands on your knees. Join the thumb and index finger on each hand into a ring. As always, lift and lengthen from the root of your spine to the crown of your head, and be open and relaxed in your hips and shoulders. Have your body so poised that you can begin to forget about it.

Give your breathing time to settle into a slow, steady rhythm.

At first it may be helpful to focus your mind on a single object, or a *mantra* (chant) such as *Om*, in order to calm the hurly-burly of thoughts. Choose what you wish to contemplate and imagine it clearly. Other thoughts will chatter, flap around, knock at the door. Simply observe them and let them go, bringing your mind back to the rose, the candle flame, the *mantra*; whatever you have chosen. At this stage the practice is more properly called *dharana* or concentration.

Begin with four or five minutes of concentration. You may feel cross and restless at first, but bear with it. After a while a feeling of calm and steadiness will come into those times.

Later on you may be able or want to extend the length of time for which you sit and let your mind become still without the aid of a focus of concentration to stop its fluctuations. You will be able simply to 'stand back', to detach yourself from your mind and watch the flow of thoughts until they cease.

The effect of meditation is often illustrated with the metaphor of the lake. The true self is the bottom of the lake. The life of consciousness is the many metres of water above it. We stand on the shore trying to understand our true selves, but the surface of the water is constantly disturbed by pebbles and stones thrown into the water. These are our thoughts occurring. All we can see is the ripples and disturbances caused by the thoughts. Only by stopping the splashing of thoughts into the water can we let the surface settle. Then we are able to look through the clear water onto the deep bedrock at the bottom of the lake.

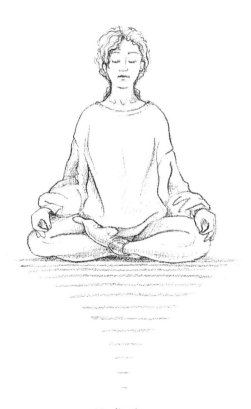

Meditation

As with *savasana*, the effect is to put us more clearly in touch with our inner strength. Most women spend large stretches of their lives with multiple commitments, remembering myriad pieces of information, some factual, some about people's emotions and feelings, and coordinating them delicately. Like an air-traffic controller bringing many aircraft safely in to land, women negotiate the complexities of career and family life, caring for parents, partners, children, maintaining health and fitness of self and family members, catering, laundering, first-aiding, counselling, and being a social secretary. A short interlude at each yoga practice of concentration or meditation, whichever is right for you, creates a wonderful sense of space in the self. Quietness spreads through body and mind, and another perspective on hectic schedules emerges, a slower, more detached, more consistent, bedrock self.

chapter three

LIFE PASSAGES

Our lives as women are marked by a series of cycles and changes as our fertility evolves and varies and changes. Our bodies change in shape and texture, lightness, heaviness, different curves and volumes coming and going. Some women remain a fairly constant size and shape throughout their lives, while others wax and wane and alter profoundly with each decade. With the ebb and flow of different hormones we experience changes in our skin and hair, our ligaments and muscle tone. We become more or less vulnerable emotionally as the cycles devolve. We are sometimes bewildered by the range of body and character which seems to consitute the entity 'myself'.

Added to this we are surrounded daily by thousands of images presenting an ideal of woman as unscathed and unchanging, tall, thin, bronzed and athletic – as well as being thin she should also have the heavy swollen breasts of a lactating mother (so much for the collective unconscious of the tabloid press), and look passive and young. Women's magazines are deeply confused over this issue, publishing regular features about eating disorders, 'body fascism' (the compulsion for everybody to undertake some sort of fitness régime), and accepting and loving one's body for what it is, while continuing to use models who reflect no such variety or broadness of vision, and continue to pile on the pressure to women to conform to one of these 'ideal' images.

Any woman who thinks about her body, its phases and changes, and her own views and emotions about it, may well find herself involved in a struggle with all kinds of contradictions. She may know that she feels comfortable and healthy at one weight, but more powerful and sexual as she moves around in society at another, much lower, weight. She may have fantasies about radical/magical plastic surgery that would make her breasts bigger or smaller or change their shape, or carve layers away from hips or ankles. Few women escape the sense of having an 'unfavourite' part of their bodies. Few women contemplate the prospect of the changes age will bring without some misgivings.

Any woman who also sees herself as a rational person, or a feminist person, or someone committed to holistic thinking, will suffer, in addition to this, a sense of stupidity and guilt, as though she ought to be able simply to decide not to feel such things.

We are looking, perhaps, for a way to live with our physical bodies at their own comfortable, healthy sizes and shapes in all the range and variety which that implies, to be strong and fit and change and age with dignity and without denial. Yoga offers a medium through which those things can begin to happen. Because the body is strengthened, opened and challenged by the postures in an appropriate way, it becomes, as it were, *more* itself, more characteristic of itself, more true to itself. The sense of tuning in to a deep level of self which develops through centring at the beginning of a practice, through the practice of *savasana* (corpse or relaxation pose), and through spending time in concentration and meditation, can be a very steadying element when there is a great deal of physical and emotional fluctuation on the surface of our lives. It may be that the steady feeling is to do with contacting an unchanging core in the centre of ourselves, or to do with an unchanging quality in the sense of peace itself.

If the phase of womanhood which you are going through feels important to you at the moment, you may like to build a yoga programme with that in mind. Remember to evolve a programme which begins with some calm time to come to centre, and ends with plenty of time with *savasana*. In the standing part of your programme include postures with strong forward and sideways stretches, and a balance to align your central upward strength. Include some appropriate back bends, sitting postures with the legs straight in front, with the legs stretched apart, and with the thighs rotated the other way (hero pose, page 31, and related postures). Programme in at least one of the many twists and, if appropriate, an upside down posture as well. You may want to do some breathing exercises, and some work with meditation too. *Savasana* closes your practice.

The poses in this chapter may feel useful to illustrate and explore various life passages. Weave them into the basic shape of your programme if they attract you. Choose intuitively, be ready to reject anything that looks and feels too stressful or in any way awkward in relation to the way your body feels, and to choose anything, from whatever section, that seems to contain a movement, an expansion, or a mood that you need. Use the whole chapter as a resource to increase your vocabulary of asanas and as a stimulus to thinking more about what each posture means to and does for you.

Remember that these postures are not compulsory, nor are they a complete programme; they must be integrated into a full and balanced programme. Choose carefully and responsibly for yourself.

ADOLESCENCE

Somewhere between eight and sixteen years of age the body of a little girl metamorphoses into that of a young woman. The date of the menarche (the beginning of menstrual periods) gets steadily younger and younger in the modern West. This seems to be to do with high levels of nutrition, and some research has also linked it with our extensive use of artificial light in the evenings: apparently one of the triggers for the release of hormones is the numbers of hours of light that have been experienced.

This poses girls who are very young in social terms with the task of coping with periods, with their own sexuality, and with other people's reactions to it.

In a matter of months they may change completely in body shape from the straight, lithe lines of a little girl, to the curves and heavier volumes of maturity. While the monthly cycle of hormonal changes settles down, there is a tendency towards the moodiness and rawness which adults find so exasperating. The adolescent person finds it exasperating too. Once we have left adolescence behind, we are extremely insulting about it – describing someone's behaviour or emotions as 'adolescent' is almost always a put-down. This is hardly fair, and perhaps comes from one's own unresolved adolescent conflicts, still unexpectedly present during every other phase of our lives. One confidently expects on arriving at one's twenties or at the latest thirties, to be adult, competent and mature, and is shocked to find that in many respects one has not changed much since one was seventeen. Perhaps this is part of the strong reaction against all things 'adolescent'.

Practice of yoga can certainly help the condition of skin and hair, the steadying of moods, the steadying of the menstrual cycle. It can also provide a way of becoming more familiar with and sensitive to new body shapes, new axes and new strengths.

You may like to include these three poses in your practice.

HANUMANASANA – MONKEY POSE

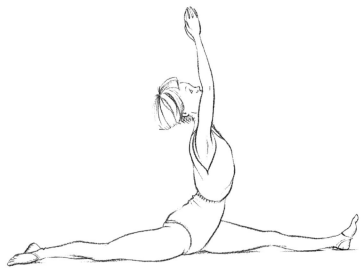

Hanumanasana (monkey pose) with arms overhead

Hanuman is the name of a strong and powerful monkey. He leapt across the sea with a huge stride bringing healing herbs to a dying warrior. This pose represents the leap of *Hanuman*.

It is a pleasant pose to practise, thinking of leaping from one phase of life to another, as powerful and agile as the monkey *Hanuman*. It is also a lovely stretch which, if you become familiar and comfortable with it while fairly young, will not come to seem a distant impossibility (which is the way it feels to people who do not try it out first until their twenties or thirties).

Warm up the fronts of your thighs first. Place your hands flat on the floor, hip distance apart, and place your right foot between your hands, bending your right knee. Slide your left leg out straight behind you, firstly with your toes tucked under, then with the top of your instep on the floor. Make sure that your left knee is facing the floor, and your left leg is stretching out straight behind you, and not veering out at an angle to the left. Feel the left leg ease out and elongate.

Now do the same thing to the other side, with your left foot between your hands, left knee bent, and your right leg stretching out behind you.

When both legs and hips have been warmed up, begin again with your right foot between your hands. Stretch your left leg out behind you, top of the instep towards the floor. Taking much of your weight on your hands, begin carefully to extend your right leg out in front of you. Do not bounce or force your leg, just go to the right place for you for now.

At first it is necessary to keep your balance and support much of your weight with your hands. As your legs and hips become more flexible you will gradually become able to sit down into your hips.

Keep your spine stretching upwards, and your neck long and supple, your shoulders loose and relaxed. Do not let the intensity of the stretch cause you to contort your face!

When you can sit without stress down in *hanumanasana*, try bringing your hands together in front of your chest in *namaste*, and when that becomes easy, stretch both arms up and join your palms high above your head. Do not let your shoulders hunch up.

Bring lightness and life to the pose by visualizing the leap. You have probably seen dancers leap across the stage like this, as though they were flying. Try to bring that feeling into your body.

Come out of *hanumanasana* slowly, taking your hands to the floor and taking some of your weight on them, and bring your front leg back gradually. Now practise the pose with equal concentration and an equal amount of time with the left leg in front and the right extended out behind.

If you continue to do this pose a few times a week you will not lose it. If you come to the pose very stiff or later on in your life, do not be disheartened by the apparent hopelessness of finding the stretch. Fit it into your life several times a week and you will be amazed to see your own progress.

UTTANA PADASANA – POSE OF TRANQUILITY

Lie on your back on the floor, making sure that your centre line is straight. Breathe steadily. On an exhalation, arch your upper back and rest the crown of your head on the floor. Take two or three steady breaths in this position and then on another exhalation, lift your legs, keeping them straight, until they are at an angle of about forty-five degrees to the floor. Raise your arms, placing your palms together, so that your arms are parallel to your legs. Feel your abdomen is strong and your chest free and open. You are balanced on the crown of your head and your buttocks.

When you want to come out of the stretch, breathing out, lower your legs and arms and, lengthening your spine and the back of your neck, lower down until you are lying flat again. If you feel tight in the back of your waist, hug your knees up onto your chest, and rock gently from side to side.

VRSCHIKASANA – SCORPION POSE

The scorpion is an exciting pose which, again, is pleasant to learn when you are young, and keep in your 'vocabulary' as you grow older.

It is a balance with a back bend incorporated in it. It feels different as your breasts and hips get heavier, but helps to give a feeling that although your body is getting larger and heavier it need not weigh you down.

Begin learning the pose with the help of a friend, a wall, and a blanket.

Fold your blanket into a pad and place it next to the wall, to make a softer landing for your face if you should come down more quickly than you intend.

Kneel on the floor close to and facing the wall and rest your elbows on the floor shoulder distance apart. Then lay your forearms on the floor parallel to one another, with your fingers pointing

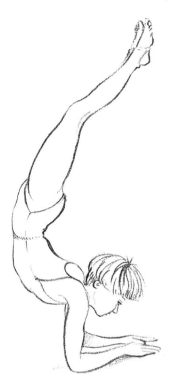

Vrschikasana (scorpion pose)

forwards. Your blanket pad is between your forearms, and there is room for your head to move forwards some way without coming into contact with the wall. Visualize your forearms as the long 'feet' you are going to balance on.

Firstly, hang your head forwards for a few seconds to lengthen and relax your neck and open your shoulders, then lift your head and move it forwards so that your chest moves forwards a little.

Exhaling, straighten your legs and stretch your hips into the air. Come up onto tiptoes to lift your hips higher, then relax your feet, so that your legs lengthen and your hips stay lifted.

Your friend should stay close to you to catch or stabilize you if you lose your balance.

On your first few attempts simply try to straighten first one leg, then the other, stretching them up into the air behind you one at a time, while keeping the other foot on the floor.

When you begin to feel accustomed to this, stretch one leg up behind you, then ask your friend to help you to bring it up till the foot rests against the wall. The other leg will naturally follow it up, and your assistant can rest the other foot against the wall too. Your assistant remains close to help you if you feel unstable, and to help you to bring your legs down again with control until you are able to manage this unassisted. Keep your whole body alert and alive. Do not flop your weight onto the soles of your feet, use your whole body strength to keep yourself there. A few seconds will be plenty at first.

When your partner has helped you to bring your legs down, sit back on your heels, and then rest forwards in the pose of the child (see page 54).

You will eventually be able to move up and down into the pose without help, then rest just your toes on the wall, and finally work in the pose in free space.

Never rush it, always collect your thoughts before you begin, and always relax in the pose of the child when you have finished.

When one achieves competence in a spectacular pose it is tempting to display it as a party piece. Of course it is a positive thing to share your exhilaration about a strong pose with friends, but bear in mind two things: firstly, that if you do not warm up properly you will probably injure yourself; and secondly that, if you intimidate rather than inspire your friends you will, in a more subtle way, injure them – so be aware of those two factors whenever you choose to show anyone any yoga poses.

MENSTRUAL CYCLE

The menstrual cycle generates an ebb and flow of hormones, an ebb and flow of energies and moods, throughout the fertile part of our life. Women who spend an extended time taking the contraceptive pill are having a different kind of cycle, and may find it useful to be aware that when they stop the pill and fertile cycles begin again, they may find them surprisingly strong. One gradually becomes accustomed to them again, but they do at first feel very different.

The suppleness and strength from practising yoga help

tremendously in flowing with the cycle rather than tensing up against it. Both posture and relaxation exercises also help with the cramps commonly experienced on the first couple of days of the period itself (but remember not to practise inverted postures during a period). In general, positive feelings about inhabiting your body and enjoying its functions make it more possible to move through this cyclic experience cheerfully. One need not attempt to pretend it is always pleasant, but it has its positive aspects. A sense of integration and concurrence with the natural world is also an important part of yoga: many of the postures are named after animals, plants, or natural objects like the mountains or the moon and in practising the pose you identify with that part of creation. Your growing awarenss of your own physical structure and mass makes you feel more clearly part of the physical material of the universe, and less like an isolated organism in a world existing only like a technicolour movie in your own head. In those terms it is easier to feel and understand the repetitions of ovulation, fullness and bleeding.

These four postures may be useful for taking into your practice during menstruation, or the week before menstruation if that is a time when you feel full or bloated or very aware of your body in a different way, or any other time when your menstrual cycle is on your mind for any reason.

PADMASANA – LOTUS POSE

The lotus has its roots in the mud, its stem in the water, and its beautiful flower in the sun. It reminds us that that is how we too can be – our roots are firmly in the mud, but we have the potential to flower out into the fresh air.

The quality of this pose is having a steady, firmly spread base, open and uncongested hips and an upward lifting, free-breathing sensation in the upper body. The lotus flower is imagined where your halo would be (*sahasraha chakra* – see page 127). The pose helps to relieve swollen feelings in the pelvis and to lengthen the whole body which tends to contract forwards a little if you are either bloated or in pain. The steadiness of the base helps to 'ground' and stabilize the emotions.

Begin *padmasana* by sitting in *dandasana*, well onto the centre of your pelvic floor, legs straight out in front and spine lifting,

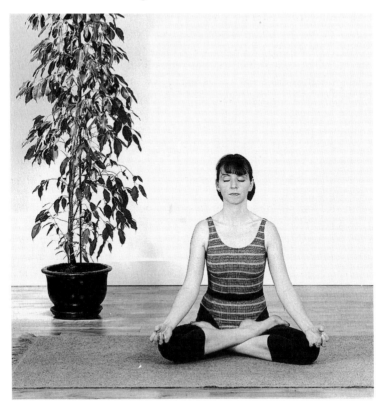

Padmasana (lotus pose)

shoulders released, neck long. Your hands are palms downwards on the floor next to your hips, fingers pointing forwards. It is better to have your elbows a little bent than to have your shoulders hunched into your ears.

Start to explore how much of *padmasana* is possible for you today. Bend your right leg, and see if you can rest the top of your right instep on top of your left thigh. If not, bring your right foot close into your perineum, and gradually turn your foot over so that you can see the sole of your right foot. Soon your knee and foot will loosen enough to bring your foot onto your opposite thigh.

If your right leg is relaxed with your foot on your left thigh, bend your left leg and bring it in to a cross-legged position: you are now in the half-lotus position. Carefully try lifting your left foot onto your right thigh. If it will rest onto your right thigh without any feeling of emergency in knee or ankle, leave it there: this is full lotus. Lift and align your spine, feel your hips becoming more and more open, and either rest your hands one cupped in the other in your lap, or the backs of your hands out onto your knees. Breathe steadily and think of the lotus.

If your foot or knee feel too uncomfortable in full lotus, move back into half lotus; if that feels stressful, have your left leg straight and right leg bent in close to the body. When you feel ready to, come out of lotus pose by carefully untangling your legs, and return to *dandasana*.

Spend an equal amount of time with the pose beginning on the other side of the body so that the left leg bends first, and come carefully out of the pose on this side too, returning to *dandasana*.

If you have uncomfortable cramps it is helpful to go into a forward bend from the full lotus position, so that your feet are pressing into the pelvic area, counteracting the tension of the cramp. Remember to inhale and extend your torso upwards before you exhale and stretch forwards. A variation which is useful if full lotus is not comfortable for you, is to sit cross-legged, make loose fists with your hands and rest them low down on the abdomen, and then to stretch your upper body forwards and down – your fists will press into the area of the cramp and relax it somewhat.

URDHVA DHANURASANA – BRIDGE POSE

Urdhva dhanurasana is the position which, as children, we called 'crab'. It is a lovely position for relieving a bloated feeling of the abdomen, because it gives a long, strong stretch to the front of the body, while arching your spine in a powerful back bend. It also brings a sense of strength and confidence.

Begin by lying on your back with your knees bent and feet flat on the floor, then rest your hands on the floor bent back (fingers pointing towards your feet) at shoulder level. You may need to spend some time becoming accustomed to this hand position.

When you feel ready, come up onto the crown of your head. Stay in this position until you feel prepared to exhale and lift up onto hands and feet, your arms and legs strong, and breathe steadily. A few seconds will be plenty at first, but as time goes on you will be

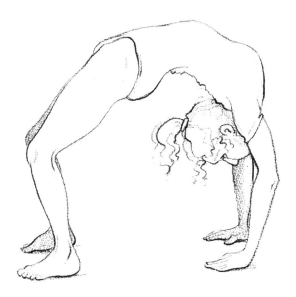

Urdhva dhanurasana (bridge pose)

able to stay up longer, up to half a minute or so. Enjoy the feeling of the back bend, and of the front surface of your body being opened and stretched.

When you want to come down, lift your head a little, and with your neck long, unwind your spine slowly and with control onto the floor. When your hips reach the floor, think of your lower back spreading out. Hug your knees onto your chest and rock gently from side to side.

Your wrists and forearms may feel ridiculously weak at first. Think of strength flowing up from under the floor into your arms, up and over, and down into your legs and feet. Your hands and arms will soon feel stronger.

When *urdhva dhanurasana* becomes easy you can try some variations: take your chest and head back a little over your hands and arms, and walk your feet together, then out until your legs are straight; or carefully move one foot into a central position, inhale and lift the other knee to your chest, then exhale and stretch the leg straight up. Bring it down by bending the knee again and placing your foot to the floor, then repeat it to the other side.

ARDHA CHANDRASANA - HALF MOON POSE

People who work or travel at night, or live in the country away from artificial night lighting, become aware of the phases of the moon. We are missing out when we live a life when we no longer see the moon or know whether it is waxing, full, or waning. If you start to look out for the moon you can see where your own cycle fits with the moon's.

Many diaries have a menstrual calendar which will show how your particular rhythm ripples across the months.

The half moon pose is triangle pose, *trikonasana*, extended out into a balance. You can try it first with your back against a wall for support, and progress to performing the pose in free space.

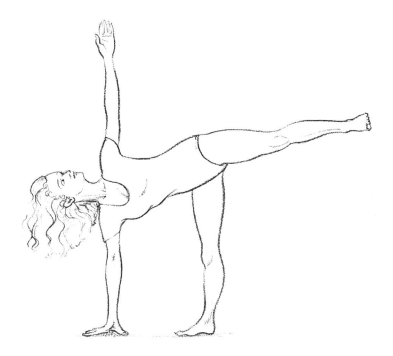

Ardha chandrasana (half moon pose)

Being careful to extend your lower waist fully, move into *trikonasana* (see page 26).

Turn to look at your front foot. Inhale, and lay your upper arm along the top edge of your waist. As you exhale, bend your front knee, place your front hand on the floor a foot or so in front of your front foot, straighten your front leg as you lift your straight back leg and push your heel away. Breathe steadily.

If you feel secure, turn your gaze to the front and focus on some particular point. When you are stable, stretch your upper arm straight up into the air, palm forwards. Your whole body is open, stretched, and poised. Be aware of your face, keep it serene! Do not let your concentration cause you to clench your teeth or crease your brow.

When you want to come down, come back into *trikonasana*, and then stand up on an inhalation and lower your arms on the exhalation.

Work equally on *ardha chandrasana* on the other side.

CHATAKASANA – SKYLARK POSE

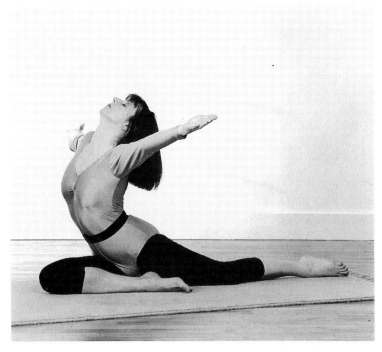

Chatakasana (skylark pose)

This beautiful pose gives a feeling of lightness – a marvellous way to balance any sense of sluggishness or heaviness. If you have practised *hanumanasana* you will not find it difficult.

Fit *chatakasana* into your session after *hanumanasana* (page 62) and *bhujangasana* (page 39), as these will warm up and loosen your thighs, hips, and back.

Begin with your hands on the floor, hip distance apart, your right knee bent and your right foot between your hands.

Ease your left leg out behind you, the top of your instep on the floor, knee facing downwards. Be careful that your left leg is stretching straight out behind you, and not veering to the left or right.

Bring your bent right knee to the ground and tuck your right foot into your perineum. Balance with your fingertips on the floor on either side of your hips.

When you feel ready, take a breath in, then exhale stretching your spine up and back, stretching your arms out, hands palm up, at shoulder level. Breathe steadily.

Enjoy the exhilaration of this pose, before carefully exhaling and coming back to a relaxed cross-legged position until your breathing and heartbeat have settled down again and you are ready to do *chatakasana* with your other leg in front.

PREGNANCY

During the first three months of an uncomplicated pregnancy you can practise all your normal postures as the baby is still tucked down into your pelvis. However, if you do ever feel stressed, come gently out of the posture and rest in *savasana* or lying on your side (see page 79) until you feel comfortable again. If you have had bleeding or any other difficulties, discuss with your midwife when it would be safe and advisable for you to begin doing yoga again. Take your yoga book with you to show them the stretches you would like to do if you think they may not be familiar with yoga poses.

After twelve weeks or so you will feel the fundus (the top of the uterus) gradually rising up into the abdomen. There are a few postures which should be avoided once this starts to happen: firstly anything which involves lying on your tummy on the floor (such as

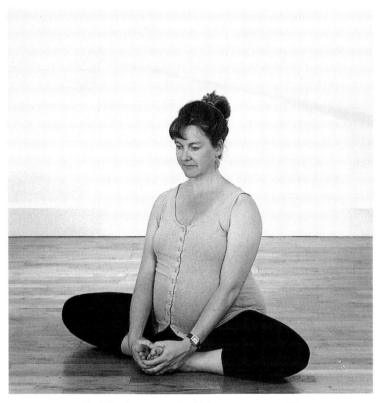

Baddha konasana (cobbler pose, page 47)
in eighth month of pregnancy

cobra, or locust); secondly, strong back bends (like *urdhva dhanurasana* and, unless you are very confident in it, *ustrasana*), and any twisting postures which make your abdomen feel squashed. Unless you have practised for several years, or are working with an experienced teacher, avoid inverted postures, by doing dog pose (no. 8 in *surya namaskar,* page 110) and modified headstand (head and arms in position, hips up, feet on floor) instead.

Be attentive to your body and avoid anything which feels forced or wrong. As your abdomen grows, be aware that your centre of gravity will change and your balance will be different, particularly in poses like *trikonasana.*

The joy of yoga in pregnancy is the opportunity to enjoy your changing shape and swelling curves, while remaining graceful and powerful. The stretching and mobility help to relieve back and shoulder aches, and to expand and strengthen the pelvic outlet and the pelvic floor. Both *savasana* and meditation are a chance to reflect on the miracle of the small life growing gradually to independence inside you.

SQUATTING POSE

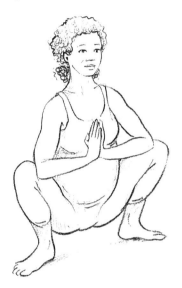

Squatting pose   Modified squatting pose

This comfortable and relaxing posture becomes alien to us when we sit on chairs and wear high-heeled shoes, and we lose the lovely flexion and opening in our hips.

You may need to begin to relearn squatting with your heels resting on a thick book (a dictionary or phone book would be useful) and your elbows resting loosely on your knees.

Gradually decrease the height of the lift under your heels as the weeks go by, and you will eventually find your heels resting comfortably on the floor.

Also, case your elbows in-between your knees and press your palms together, levering your thighs wider apart.

Work on lengthening your neck and spine, and also lengthening the front of your body so that it does not feel bundled or crumpled up.

Once you are fully at ease in a squat you may like to begin standing up straight with your feet a couple of feet apart, toes turned slightly out, then place your palms together, and on an exhalation, bend your knees, and flow down into a full squat, elbows between your knees, spine upright.

Remain in the squat for half a minute at first, longer later.

If you look at yourself in a studio mirror while squatting, or look at somebody else in a squatting position, you will see the beautiful opening of the hips, and the pelvic floor spread right out. This extra stretch and space will ease your baby's delivery.

If your legs feel strong and sure, come out of the squat by exhaling, pressing your feet into the floor, and lengthening and straightening your legs to stand up.

Otherwise, reach forwards to rest a hand on the floor, and put your knees onto the floor to come out of the stretch.

Frog pose and pelvic floor exercise

Kneel with your feet together, and your knees wide apart. If your bottom will not yet rest onto your heels, just go back as far as is comfortable. If your knees feel very tight or stressed, put a couple of cushions or pillows under your hips until you feel more flexible.

Inhaling, lift your head and stretch your spine up and, exhaling, walk your hands forwards along the floor. At your comfortable maximum, relax your head and neck down. Make sure you are lengthening, and not compressing, the front of your body. As the weeks pass, the floor gets nearer.

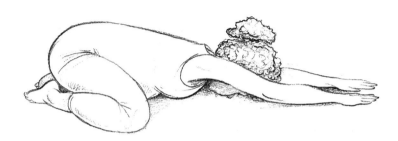

Frog pose

When you have extended into the pose of the frog, focus on your pelvic floor muscles. If you aren't sure where these are, imagine that you need to go to the toilet, but that there is no toilet available nearby. Contract the muscles that you would need to contract in that situation – a ring of muscles around the front passage, and another ring around the back passage, arranged together like a figure of eight. At first you may find you can hardly cause the muscles to contract voluntarily at all, but it is very important to learn to strengthen these muscles, so persevere.

Squeeze and release your pelvic floor muscles half a dozen times when you are in the frog pose, then breathe in and lift your head, exhale and walk your hands towards you to come up.

Frog pose opens the hips and thighs, and also gives a sense of stretching and opening to the lower back which helps to alleviate the tender backache that arises because of the softening of ligaments caused by hormonal changes. This softening will often make your poses more open and extended during pregnancy, and you will find that so long as you practise fairly steadily, you can carry that extra stretch and movement with you when the pregnancy is over. The softening does, however, mean that you should treat your joints with extra respect and, particularly, never be tempted to bounce limbs or joints in order to increase your stretch.

When you kneel or stand up, take your thoughts once more to your pelvic floor muscles. You will observe that they are in roughly the area that a sanitary towel would cover. Think about what they are doing and you will realize, once you are vertical, that they are what hold your insides in! During pregnancy they also hold in several pounds of baby, placenta, liquor and membranes as well. Clearly it is important to keep these muscles in good condition, and doing so will help to prevent incontinence and prolapse later on. On the positive side, once you are aware of and in touch with these muscles, you will be more able to release and relax them when the baby is born, and your vaginal muscle tone will improve more quickly after the birth. Every time it crosses your mind, squeeze and release your pelvic floor half a dozen times.

ANJANEYASANA - CRESCENT MOON POSE

When it is no longer possible to get down onto your tummy and practise cobra, you will probably find yourself longing for a good

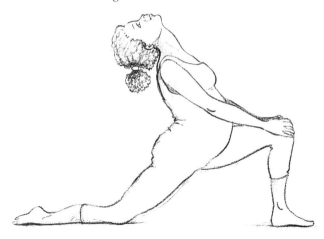

Anjaneyasana (crescent moon pose)

back bend. *Anjaneyasana*, in a modified version as in the illustration, may provide you with one.

Kneel with your left knee on the floor and your right foot on the floor, with your right knee bent. Make sure your body is facing fully to the front, and not turned at an angle.

Place your hands on your front knee to steady yourself, then stretch your left leg a little way further back, stretching the front of your left thigh and beginning the bending movement in your lower back. Keep your left knee facing the floor and your hips and chest facing the front. Breathing in, stretch your spine upwards and grow taller, being careful to keep your shoulders and your face soft. As you exhale, begin to bend your lengthened spine backwards, only as far as it feels right for you, then at your comfortable maximum take your head back, by lengthening your throat rather than by compressing your neck. Breathe steadily. When you want to come out of the pose, inhale and lift your head and, exhaling, come up. Rest forwards into the pose of the child (with your knees separated to accommodate the baby), and feel your lower back spread out and relax.

Practise *anjaneyasana* to the other side, and rest in pose of the child again afterwards.

If your head feels uncomfortably heavy in this position, or your balance becomes difficult to maintain as your baby grows inside you, you could change to the simple cat stretch exercise to mobilize your back: on all fours slowly arch and flatten your back half a dozen times in the rhythm of your own breathing. This does not of course give a backwards back bend, but will keep your spine flexible until the baby is born and you can return to the ordinary back bending positions.

ABDOMINAL BREATHING AND MODIFIED *SAVASANA*

Abdominal breathing as described in Chapter 2 (pages 53–4) is an invaluable way of calming down during pregnancy. This steady breath combined, when it becomes necessary, with a swaying movement of the hips, in any position where your hips are relaxed and open and your torso is inclined forwards in relation to your hips (this helps to open your pelvis), can help to carry you through your contractions in the first stage of labour.

In the later months of pregnancy, if you become heavy and weary, you may like to practise both abdominal breathing and *savasana*, lying on your side.

Choose your left side, because then your heavy uterus is not pressing onto your vena cava, the major vessel returning blood to your heart. The vena cava runs along the right-hand side of the spinal column, so by lying on the left side, you are rolling the weight of the uterus away from it. Have a cushion or pillow under your head, and another under your bent right knee, and make your arms comfortable either by sliding your left arm out under you to your left side, or if your breasts are too sore for this, by curling your arms loosely into a foetal position, keeping your shoulders and chest as loose and open as you can.

Do a few cycles of abdominal breathing, then allow your breath to settle where it wants to: it will probably be slow and light. Now rest in *savasana*, muscles and joints heavy and soft, face and throat soft, back soft and spreading out, feet and hands warm and heavy.

After some time in *savasana* you may feel you want to put a hand onto your abdomen and say hello to the baby.

The baby may sometimes swim over and push back onto your hand! This pre-birth communication comes naturally to many mothers and many babies, and is a happy beginning to your relationship with one another.

Remember that the poses suggested here are not a complete

sequence for pregnancy, but should be fitted into a full and balanced programme as we have described. Do not hesitate to redesign your programme every 5 or 6 weeks during pregnancy to reflect your body's different shape and different needs, and do not be afraid to concentrate more on the sitting poses in the last few weeks if you are tired. Sometimes our modern culture's dictum that, as a woman, you should be fit, thin, and sexually available every moment of your life leaves your ability to work out how you feel and what you want (let alone how to get it) in shreds. Is it lazy, will you be gross and slothful if you only or primarily do floor poses in the last weeks of pregnancy? Of course not. What is right for you today? Choose that. Do not feel inadequate if you are not sure what it is – most of our conditioning and education has prompted us to think that what our own impulse is will probably be wrong. Just sit with it until it becomes clear to you what it is. Do not be afraid to be sometimes large and sometimes small, to be sometimes strong and sometimes weak, sometimes fast and sometimes slow.

> To every thing there is a season, and a time to
> every purpose under the heaven:
> A time to be born, and a time to die; a time to
> plant, and a time to pluck up that which is planted;
> A time to kill, and a time to heal; a time to break
> down and a time to build up;
> A time to weep and a time to laugh; a time to mourn
> and a time to dance; . . .
> A time to get and a time to lose, a time to keep
> and a time to cast away; . . .
> A time to love, and a time to hate; a time of war,
> and a time of peace . . .
>
> *Ecclesiastes* 3:1

This is echoed in Lao Tzu:

> For all things there is a time for going ahead, and a
> time for following behind,
> A time for slow breathing, and a time for fast breathing,
> A time to grow in strength and a time to decay,
> A time to be up and a time to be down.
> Therefore the sage avoids all extremes, excesses,
> and extravagances.

Not every woman is or should be an athlete right through her pregnancy. What we can do for each other is to accept and celebrate the whole spectrum of shape, fitness and frame of mind in each of us at this special time.

THE POST-NATAL MONTHS

Psychologists tell us that new mothers are involved in something called 'primary preoccupation' with their babies. New mothers of course know that their primary preoccupation is with getting enough sleep! Actually, of course the involvement with the new baby is, in turns, exciting, heartrendingly tender, tedious, frustrating, delightful, all manner of contradictory qualities simultaneously and this is, therefore, a demanding time for the woman. Many of us undertake without the support of an extended family the months of learning to live with a new, and initially very dependent little person, often with little sleep and a cut in income and social recognition. (For all the lip service our society pays to 'family values', women caring for children are often, astonishingly, described as 'not working'.) We are also perhaps learning the art of breastfeeding, trying to work out a new identity for ourselves and trying to rest, heal, and restrengthen our bodies.

Many women are preoccupied too with when they might be able to get back into their ordinary clothes again, and the change from the magnificent fullness of 9 months of pregnancy, to a shape which is much larger than you were before you became pregnant can be a great shock. Patience is really the answer. If you are not one of the (very few) women who revert immediately to their pre-pregnant shape, do not panic and do not hate your body. Its capacity for change and recovery is tremendous, and you can be well-toned and have a defined shape again, it simply takes time. (One woman, who always looked pretty slim to me, confided, 'It was 16 weeks after the birth before I could get my jeans past my *knees*.')

You can begin doing postures gently any time you feel like it after 2 weeks post-delivery. (If you had a Caesarean section you will want to leave it a few weeks longer.) Do not do inverted postures while you are still losing lochia (the post-natal bleeding). If you notice that your bleeding gets heavier during or after doing postures, or indeed during or after any activity, it indicates that you are overdoing things, and should rest more.

Begin by attempting perhaps five or six postures at the most, per day, and gradually increase the length of the programme during the following weeks, as you grow stronger.

Good quality rest during the weeks after the birth of a baby is more valuable than money in the bank. At any interlude or opportunity, have a few minutes of *savasana*, or abdominal breathing, or quiet meditation. You can conserve energy and reach your deep inner core of strength by doing so.

You will enjoy your new lightness when you remake your programme again, though do watch your balance in the standing poses, as your centre of gravity is, yet again, different from how it was before the baby was born. You may like to incorporate some of these postures into your programme. Go gently, the hormones which loosened your ligaments and joints during pregnancy may still be circulating in your body up to six months after the birth.

MATSAYASANA - FISH POSE

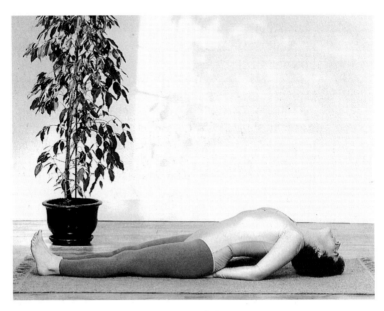

Matsayasana (fish pose)

Matsayasana can come into your practice as a back bend. It is also a useful counter-posture to follow shoulder stand, taking any residual tension out of the neck and shoulders. It is named after Matsya, the fish, one of the forms taken by the god Vishnu, who took on this shape in order to save the world from the Flood.

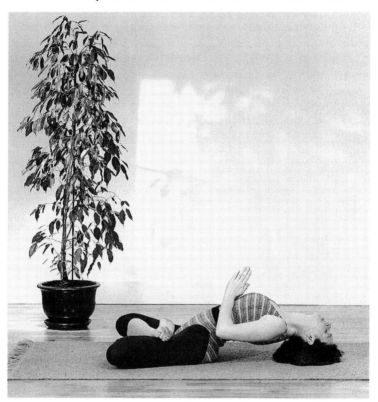

Matsayana in *padmasana* (fish pose in lotus pose)

Try the milder form of this pose first. Lie on your back, with the centre line of your body straight. Place your hands palms down, under your hips. Have your hands as close together as you can, and slide them down as far towards your thighs as you can.

On an exhalation, press your elbows into the ground, arch your upper back, and come up onto the crown of your head. Lengthen all along your legs and stretch your heels away so that your toes point up towards the ceiling. Breathe steadily. Keep your elbows close together underneath your shoulders, and keep your chest open and your shoulders soft.

To come out of *matsayasana*, inhale and lift your head gently, then lay it on the ground, slide your arms out from underneath you and rest.

If you are comfortable in *padmasana*, the lotus, you can move into *matsayasana* by leaning back onto your elbows, then bringing the crown of your head back onto the floor. Press your palms together above your heart.

Come out of the posture by pushing up onto your elbows again. Don't forget, when you have had a rest, to recross your legs into *padmasana* with the other foot on top, and repeat the posture.

JANU SIRSASANA - SEATED FORWARD STRETCH

This can be included as a forward bend.

Begin in *dandasana*. Bring your left heel into your perineum and open your left hip and knee out to the side. Reach behind you to feel whether your hips are still level (it is easy accidentally to shoot the straight leg hip forwards). If your bent knee feels stressed, support it on a folded blanket or cushion while your hip becomes more accustomed to opening.

Inhale and stretch up out of your hips, stretch both arms straight up into the air: make a stretch that comes from your base on the ground right up through to your fingertips – not a stretch just from the armpits up.

On your exhalation stretch forwards and then down, to your comfortable maximum, holding onto your leg or foot wherever is convenient for you and emphasizing a forward movement with a lengthened spine, rather than a downward movement with a curved spine. Keep your neck lengthened and soft.

To come up, exhale and lift your spine up to the vertical all in one piece, with a broad, flat back. Repeat *janu sirsasana* to the other side.

ANANTASANA - WHEEL POSE

Anantasana is named after the serpent from whose centre the lotus grew. It represents the wheel of creativity. It is an appropriate pose for this moment in your life. You have joined in creating a new baby, you are engaged in creating a new family, and you are also creating a new identity and place in the world for yourself: and that is apart from perhaps creating breast milk, a constant stream of meals and laundry and a pleasant environment for your family, and on top of that any other projects you might have.

Anantasana is a combination between a tricky balance and an intense stretch – as a new mother you are familiar with the feeling!

It also helps to maintain the extra stretch and openness of hips and thighs which you will have developed if you practised yoga during your pregnancy.

Begin by lying on your side and looking along the floor to make sure you are lying in a straight line.

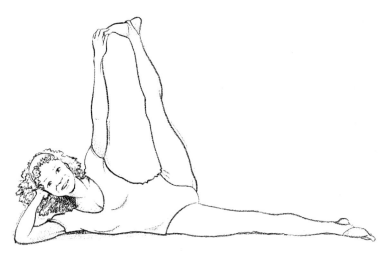

Anantasana (wheel pose)

Since there is a balancing element to this posture, look straight ahead, and choose where you will settle your gaze when you have extended into the pose. Rest your lower elbow on the floor, and your head on your hand, but do not collapse into your lower shoulder.

Bend your upper knee up towards your ear, and with your upper arm in front of the leg grasp your big toe with your second and third fingers.

If that is as far as you want to go today, that's fine. Steady your gaze, breathe steadily, and become accustomed to the balance. As you can feel, this posture strengthens the upper body as well as opening the hips and legs.

When you are ready to take the posture further, on an exhalation start to straighten your upper leg. Almost inevitably your hips will begin to tip backwards. Be aware of this and work to keep your hip vertical, as vertical as your shoulder girdle lifting from the floor. Eventually you will be able to combine a straight upper leg with keeping your hips open and upright, and your upper body poised and strong.

If you should topple over backwards, bend your knees so that you fall safely and do not hurt your back. Get your breath back and try again.

Breathe steadily in *anantasana*, and when you want to come down, exhale bending your upper leg, release your hold and stretch your upper leg straight out along the lower one.

Bend your knees, push your hands into the floor to lever yourself round, then lie on your other side, and repeat the pose with the other leg on top.

THE MENOPAUSE

At any time between our late thirties and our early sixties we may find ourselves in the menopause, the phase which may last anything between a few months and a couple of years, during which we move through the last part of our fertility and into a new and different time.

The menopause has had a bad press for a long time, and certainly many of us find ourselves vulnerable and confused as the physiological changes gradually reach a new equilibrium within us. Nevertheless, our lives as women have taught us well how to adapt and cope with change, and how to make and remake our lives again and again as circumstances and focus change.

Women have begun to write, speak, and share about the menopause, and this resource may be useful as we experience it. Many Well Woman Centres and Family Planning Clinics organize Menopause Groups where both the physical and emotional aspects can be discussed.

It is useful to continue with yoga – the physical activity helps us to retain muscle tone and flexibility, and to stimulate and regulate the workings of the soft inner organs. If you have practised yoga for a long time, your flexibility will be maintained. If you have only just made a beginning with yoga, work gently and remember always only to go to the right place for yourself in any of the stretches. Your body will soon feel loose and refreshed.

When menopause arises as a crisis for us it is sometimes not only the physical symptoms but also the predicament of being a woman undeniably ageing in a culture which seems only to value young women. One woman said, 'I felt marginalized as soon as I stopped being what could be very clearly classed as young and pretty.' We have a bad record of respecting and caring for any older people irrespective of gender in the modern West, so no wonder we feel apprehensive about it.

We may not be able to affect the whole culture immediately, but we can affect our own sense of ourselves, and other people's perception of us. We need to become attuned to the shape of our time on the earth and accept the ageing process as inevitable and as having its own form and dignity. This does not mean becoming depressed and decrepit, but it does mean finding out how we want to feel, move and look, and not panicking when it has its own quality which is different from how we felt, moved and looked in our twenties. Our experiences may not all be happy but they are rich and varied, and give us a depth, and a capacity for compassion.

Look out for images – photographs, news pictures, paintings, sculptures, of strong older women being themselves without fear; these will inspire you.

These poses may be useful, fitted into your basic programme.

VIRABHADRASANA I – WARRIOR POSE I

Virabhadrasana I is the first form of the warrior pose. It helps to move timidity and tentativeness out of the body, and to draw into it a feeling of power and strength. Power and strength come in many guises and in many ways. Use this pose as a chance to celebrate your own personal battles and your own personal courage, and to feel the decisiveness and strength in your whole self.

Begin in *tadasana*. Now step your feet four to four and a half feet apart. Turn your left foot in and your right foot out, right heel in line with left instep. Put your hands palm to palm together in front of your heart, in the *namaste* position.

Inhale, standing up tall. As you exhale turn your hips and chest to face in the direction of your right leg. Take another breath in as you adjust and align yourself, and then, exhaling, bend your front knee so that the shin remains vertical and the thigh, as you loosen up, gradually comes down to being parallel to the floor. Avoid shooting your knee out beyond your front foot. If you need to, let your back heel come off the floor, but keep your back knee straight.

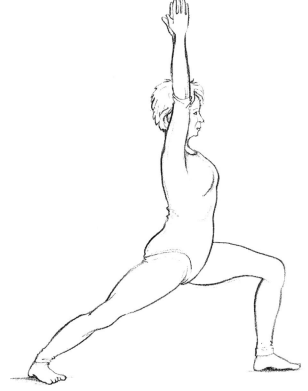

Virabhadrasana I (warrior pose I)

Breathe steadily. Let your whole self from navel level down be full of a downward flowing strength to stabilize you. From the navel level up, feel strength flowing upwards to keep your spine lifting, your head lifting, and your unstressed shoulders open and down.

This is a powerful position. A few seconds will be quite enough

at first. Later you can stay for half a minute or so. When you want
to come up, exhale fully. On the in breath press into your feet and
flow upwards to straighten your legs, then exhale to turn body and
feet to the front and relax your hands down.

Let your breathing and pulse settle before practising
virabhadrasana I to the other side.

Dragonfly pose

The pose of the dragonfly is a charming pose to look at and a
pleasant one to perform. The lower back is stretched and the
abdomen and thighs are stretched and extended. The shoulders are
working too in the completed pose. Approach the pose of the
dragonfly one step at a time and do not force your body to go farther
than it is ready to.

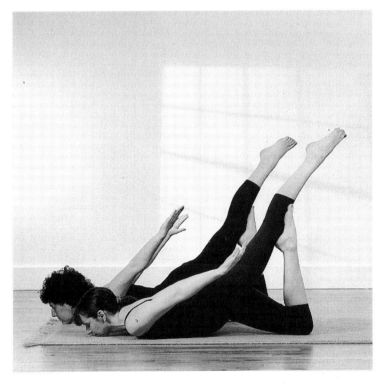

Dragonfly pose

The atmosphere of the dragonfly pose is a summery one. Allow it to remind you of pleasant picnics by lakes and streams where you have seen dragonflies hover over the water's surface. Their zooming and humming can be quite strong and alarming, but their irridescent colour and skimming flight pattern is fascinating, and their ephemeral life span a reminder of the fleeting nature of time. Once you are more deeply involved with yoga (see Chapter 6) your perspective about time changes, and this is no longer the irretrievable sadness that it was.

Begin by lying on the floor on your front – ensure that the centre line of your body is straight. At first, slide your hands palms upwards underneath the fronts of your thighs to stabilize and support your legs. Now bring your forehead to the floor. Try out bending first one knee, then the other, to check how that feels; then bend your right knee, and on a breath out straighten and stretch your left leg out and up behind you until you can rest it onto your right foot. You will find that the left knee fits comfortably into the right instep. Remain for a few seconds, breathing steadily, then on an exhalation, unbend your right leg and slowly lower down. Push up onto all fours on an in-breath, and sit back in the pose of the child on an out-breath, resting there for a few moments and visualizing your lower back spreading out, before beginning to practise the posture on the other side.

If you could not get your left leg up onto your right foot without stress, unbend the right knee a little at a time until you get to a point where you can rest your left leg onto it. Make that your place to begin, and bend the lower leg a little more each time to raise the upper leg fraction by fraction every time you try it. Remember to rest in the pose of the child, as above, before you work on the other side.

If you found the posture quite easy, try it next time with your arms alongside your body, palms towards the ceiling, then if that feels safe, progress to exhaling and stretching your arms up behind you, palms up to the ceiling as you begin. Take the stretch right into every fingertip, and feel the hovering lightness of the pose. When you want to come down, exhale and float your arms down first, then on another exhalation, with control unbend the lower knee, and lie flat out on your front. As before, inhaling, push up onto all fours and, exhaling, lengthen, sinking back onto your heels, then stretching forwards into the pose of the child. Remember to do dragonfly pose for an equal length of time on the other side.

GOMUKHASANA – COW POSE

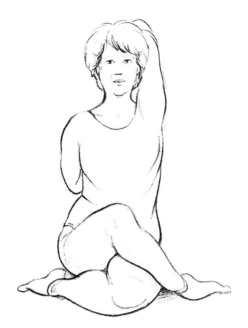

Gomukhasana (cow pose)

The name of this pose means 'the face of the cow'. Given the way in which the word 'cow' is used as an insulting name for a woman in our culture, added to the generally insulting attitude towards women travelling through the menopause ('she's at a funny age you know') you may find this a less than attractive prospect. Reflect, however, on the fact that in the culture where yoga comes from the cow is a sacred animal and her qualities of patience and stoicism along with her capacity to feed and nourish are revered. We can also usefully attempt to deprogramme ourselves and, by our influence, the people around us, from using analogies with animals in a derogatory way which is unfair both to the humans and the animals being described. This discipline of thought can be seen as a part of *ahimsa*, or non-violence (see Chapter 5), where the violence involved is a writing-off or marginalization of people or animals without a proper effort to recognize their true qualities. One woman said, with feeling, that she felt society treats the menopause as 'a kind of stupid ungainly joke, like mothers-in-law'. A woman strengthened with yoga may find it possible to experience it instead as a rite of passage to a new part of her life, different certainly, with losses certainly, but with gains as well.

The physical benefits of *gomukhasana* are an increased elasticity in the legs and knees and a full movement in the shoulders. The shoulder movement is particularly useful if tension and anxiety tend to locate themselves in your neck and shoulder area. Several variations of leg position are described; choose whichever is appropriate for you.

The classical arrangement for your legs in this pose is as in the drawing on page 91, with knees one above the other and feet tucked in. Try it cautiously, but if your knees feel tight or stressed sit instead back onto your heels or, if necessary, place a folded blanket on a cushion or pillow between your heels and kneel back onto that. If none of these is comfortable, sit cross-legged, or cross-legged with a blanket or cushions under your bottom or supporting your knees. Lift and align your spine, lift the crown of your head, lengthening the back of your neck. Relax your shoulders and feel spacious in both the front and the back of your body.

Wriggle your left arm up between your shoulder blades. Carefully reach your right hand round behind you and catch your left elbow, helping it across and thus helping your left hand further up. If you cannot yet reach your left elbow with your right hand, don't worry, just do what's right for you for today. Balance your right fingertips on the floor by your right hip. Inhaling, stretch your right arm out and then straight up, feeling the movement in your chest and shoulder. As you exhale bend your right elbow and reach your right hand down to make contact with your left. Clasp your hands or wrists together. Breathe steadily.

Maybe your left hand is miles away – if so, come slowly out of your stretch (by reversing the steps) and come into it again, this time holding a sock or a scarf (or anything else suitable) in your right hand. This will dangle down your back and you will be able to grasp the other end of it with your left hand, as time goes on working your hands closer towards each other. Keep your face soft, and your eyes large and soft like the cow's. When you wish to finish the pose, breathe in, release your hold and stretch your right arm up again and, exhaling, stretch slowly out and down, enjoying the movement. Slide your left arm down.

When you work on the other side you may be surprised at the difference, it may be markedly easier or more difficult depending on which is your usual leading side. The evening up of freedom in the shoulders which comes from regular practice of *gomukhasana* brings relaxation and evenness in the face, neck, back and even hips, by levelling up many different kinds of movements. It is useful to gradually become used to alternating the side on which you carry bags, the hip on which you carry children, the hand and arm with which you do any activities which are not so specialized that you can only manage them with your leading hand. You will feel a greater balance, loosening, strength and ease throughout your body if you do this. Notice if one of your shoulders always seems higher and tighter than the other: if so, this is the shoulder with which you try to organize the world. Imagine sending your breath to this shoulder when you do centring, *tadasana* and *dandasana*, and think of dispersing the extra concentration of tension with the breath out. Use *gomukhasana* to help this process if it's difficult to let it go.

chapter four

LIFE EVENTS

The suggestions for this chapter concern choosing extra postures to bring into your basic programme when your life is passing through particular events or emotional phases. The reasons for choosing the poses mentioned here are partly physiological and party interpretative. As with the postures in the 'Life Passages' section, these are suggestions for you to use creatively yourself. Omit any which feel inappropriate for you, and choose any that feel right even if they do not appear to match specifically with the 'life event' you are experiencing now. There may, for example, be times when you feel very alone even though apparently surrounded by people, or times when you feel a failure even though on the surface of your life you seem to be in a successful phase: and of course, the paradox could be the other way around, and although the circumstances of your life look grim, you could be feeling a real satisfaction and sense of your own strength and success in survival.

Long practice of yoga makes a subtle alteration in our emotional perspective. It is described by Eknath Easwaran in his introduction to the *Bhagavad Gita* with a rather down-to-earth simile:

When I look at a fresh, ripe, mango, it is natural for my senses to respond; that is their nature. But I should be able to stand aside and watch this interaction with detachment, the way people stand and watch while movers unload a van. In that

way I can enjoy what my senses report without ever having to act compulsively on their likes and dislikes.
The Bhagavad Gita; page 26, trans. Easwaran, Arkana, 1988

Because we value and admire passionate involvement and commitment in our culture we may initially dislike the idea of detachment. However, a sense of what is meant by detachment grows in the context of yoga: it is not a cold indifference, more a sense of being both in and out of a situation simultaneously, of intense involvement balanced by a watching and observing in a kind of compassionate detachment. This shift of attitude develops spontaneously over the months and years that we practise.

Postures in this chapter, then, can be used for celebration or comfort, or whatever you feel you need.

ALONE OR SEPARATED

We may experience isolation at many times in our lives. It may come because we are socially or geographically isolated, or financially isolated – too broke to go out, or join classes, or participate in things. We may be working with colleagues who do not seem to be on our wavelength, or perhaps there are times when nobody in our immediate family is attending to anything we think, feel, or say.

Necessity may have separated us from loved friends or partners, or they may have rejected and abandoned us. This last is perhaps the most devastating of all. The particular impact on women of broken or damaged partnerships is well described by Jean Baker Miller in her book *Towards a New Psychology of Women*:

> . . . women stay with, build on, and develop in a context of attachment to and affiliation with others. Indeed, women's sense of self [is] very much organized around being able to make and then maintain affiliation and relationships. Eventually for many women, the threat of disruption of an affiliation is perceived not as just a loss of a relationship but as something closer to a total loss of self . . .

This feeling can come too, when a loved friend or partner dies.

Thus, when we lose a loving partnership we are faced not only with remaking our lives, but, at a fundamental level, with remaking ourselves. Although it is a struggle, if you are in the middle of this at the moment, try to hold on to the fact that it is possible and will eventually happen that, although you can be bruised and miserable, the central and unique quality that makes you yourself cannot be dismantled:

> The Self cannot be pierced by weapons or burned by fire; water cannot wet it, nor can the wind dry it. The Self cannot be pierced or burned, made wet or dry. It is everlasting and infinite, standing on the motionless fountains of eternity.
>
> *Bhagavad Gita* 2:23, 24, trans. Easwaran, Arkana, 1988

'Self' here does not mean what we call 'ego', but is closer to what we might call 'soul' or 'spirit'. This is not to suggest that the pain we feel is not real and vivid, but that there is a part of ourselves that cannot be destroyed.

Sometimes we are happy to be alone, and love the sense of clarity and independence which a chosen and powerful independence brings. If parts of our life have been overcrowded we may seek out and exult in times to move freely about the world, think our own thoughts through to the end and become more familiar with our own moods and rhythms, away from the necessity of adapting to others.

TADASANA - MOUNTAIN POSE (SEE PAGE 23)

Whether or not you are alone or feeling alone by choice, and whether or not you feel positive about it, *tadasana* is an important posture.

Spend time really rooting down from beneath the soles of your feet well into the earth. Grow up through your spine and feel the crown of your head aspiring towards the sky. Feel the strength in your legs.

If you are enjoying your solitude it can be exhilarating to visualize yourself standing in *tadasana* from gradually further and further away, until you seem to see yourself as a tiny figure standing on the curved surface of the planet. You are alone but also part of the world, the gaia organism, standing on the skin of the beautiful earth.

If you feel lonely, sense what is happening in your body. It may well be that the front of your body feels crumpled and collapsed, as though you were trying to curve round your abdomen and protect it. Breathe in, and as you exhale, straighten up and make space in the front of your body – then continue to breathe steadily. You may feel a little tremulous at first, but you will soon feel stronger and braver. This applies at any time when you are feeling closed in around the front of your body because you are upset. By stretching and opening the front of your body you will feel that you literally 'lift your heart'.

Become aware of your feet on the ground and imagine that you are standing in the hard, wet sand at the edge of the sea; visualize your clear, even footprints. Now think of the earth as the mother that can sustain you, even at your most vulnerable. Think of yourself as a plant that can draw up strength through its roots. Imagine your sap rising, up through hips, chest, neck and head, along your arms and into your fingertips. Feel the new energy and potential there, know you are supple and alive. Even if you only experience that aliveness for a fleeting moment, it is enormously helpful to know it can be there.

Standing in *tadasana*, appreciate how brave you are in managing your present loneliness. Withstanding these times makes us very strong and resilient. Connect in your mind with all the other women who have ever been betrayed, abandoned or left in loneliness, and you will begin to get hold of the thread of your own survival.

PARSVAKRONASANA – SIDE FLANK STRETCH (SEE PAGE 30)

This strong sideways stretch opens your chest and hips in a powerful extension, and emphasizes strength in the thighs and calves. It helps to stop your chest and abdomen from feeling weak and caved in (as in the benefits of *tadasana* described above), and fills the lower body with life and resilience. Practise equally to each side. The increase in circulation and depth of breathing will help any feelings of numbness and alienation to disappear, and you will feel more fully present in each cell of your body.

ARDHA VIRASANA PASCHIMOTTANASANA – FORWARD STRETCH IN HALF HERO POSE

Begin in *dandasana*, then take your right leg round beside you, as in hero pose (*virasana*, page 47). If your knees feel stressed start again and try with your blanket folded into a firm block under your hips.

Breathing in, sit up tall. Stretch your spine, lengthen in the front of your body and, hinging at your hips, exhale and stretch forwards

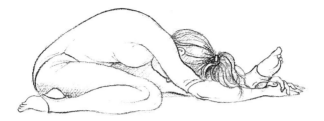

Ardha virasana paschimottanasana (forward stretch in half hero pose)

along your straight leg. Keep a feeling of moving forwards, not a feeling of moving downwards, and keep your back flat and broad. Hold onto your leg or foot wherever feels right for you, or hook a scarf round your foot and pull steadily on this to increase your stretch. After some weeks or months you will find you are lying down along your front leg.

Keep the straight leg active and alive, push your heel away and feel the stretch along the back of your leg. Notice how there is a different kind of stretch in the straight-leg hip from that in the bent-leg hip.

When you want to come up, inhale and lift your head and, exhaling, come up with a broad, flat back, and when you are all the way up remember to relax your shoulders.

Straighten your right leg out and stay for a moment in *dandasana*, before changing over and making the stretch to the other side. When you have spent a similar time in the stretch on the other side, come up carefully and gracefully and return to *dandasana*.

As well as giving a good stretch in the hips and legs, the forward bend squeezes and massages your abdomen. This, again, helps to revitalize the area of your body where you may be feeling a lot of your emotional pain.

IN A LOVING PARTNERSHIP

In the first glow of a loving partnership you may feel radiant and tingling, full of physical well-being. You will find more energy and dynamism in your stretches and have a sense of being really alive all over. As the months and years pass the first outer glow subsides but a steady inner fire may take its place.

The following postures celebrate the warmth and fulfilment of a loving partnership. They should be integrated into the balanced programme you develop for yourself.

The first two are enjoyable poses to practise with someone else. If your partner is also a yoga practitioner you may enjoy the whole range of Double Yoga poses (see Further Reading). Even if your partner
is not interested in yoga, doing the double posture with friends at class gives you a chance to explore the nuances, the meanings and the fun of bodies working and cooperating together.

DOUBLE *JANU SIRSASANA* - SHOOTING STAR POSE

Sit side by side with a partner, both in *dandasana*, with your inside legs touching. Both place your outside foot either up against your inner groin, or resting up onto the opposite thigh, as in half lotus. Making this stretch together, bring your breathing into a similar rhythm and move into the stretch gently and gradually. Look at the picture first to get a clear picture of where you are going!

Inhale and turn towards each other. Make space and an open feeling in the front of your body. Keep your hips open and loose. As

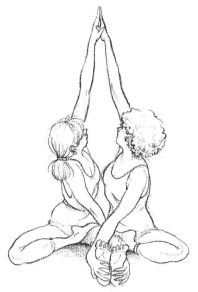

Double *janu sirsasana* (shooting star pose)

you exhale, stretch the inside arms upwards and press the palms together and, simultaneously, stretch forwards across your straight legs, as far as is a comfortable maximum for you both. When you become very loose you may eventually be able to slide your hand across your partner's ankle in order to hold the sole of her or his foot. Remain in the pose, breathing steadily, until you are ready to inhale and come up.

In order to do the pose to the other side you need to start side by side again but with the other legs touching!

The posture gives a stretching twist to the spinal column, opens the hips out, and stretches the hamstring of the straight leg.

DOUBLE *VIRASANA* - DOUBLE TREE POSE

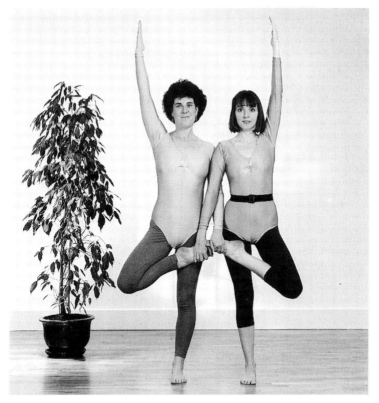

Double *virasana* (tree pose)

This pose is great fun. If your balance is too precarious to manage in free space at first, begin standing with your backs close to a wall.

You will be able to arrive at a pose like the one in the photo if your partner is a similar height to you. If not you will need to adapt, for example by stretching your outside arms out and up with palms facing in towards each other, and by the taller person putting their arm round the shorter person's shoulder, while they put their arm around the taller person's waist.

Start in *tadasana* with your adjacent feet about a foot apart. Each spread the inner foot well and get a good feeling of contact with the ground, then bring the outer foot up onto the opposite thigh, opening the bent-knee hip out as far as possible to the side, while keeping your tail bone dropping down and under and your abdomen lifted. Lift up and open through your chest, and lift up the crown of your head.

When you are ready, reach across with your inside hand and hold your partner's foot. Inhale and stretch the outside arms out and up. Either stretch the outside arms up vertically parallel or rest your palms together above your heads if you can.

Breathe rhythmically. Rest your gaze steadily on one spot in order to maintain your balance. Agree together when you are ready to exhale and disentangle yourself from the pose.

The posture stretches and strengthens the legs, opens the hips and chest, improves flexibility in the knees, and improves the balance.

Don't forget to change places and spend an equal amount of time and attention practising the pose to the other side.

When you work on yoga postures alone, you learn to observe, respect and extend your own body in fine detail. When you work with a partner you begin to extend that attention to the details of another body's scope and way of being – obviously this is a parallel to what goes on in a loving and cooperative partnership.

SETU BHANDASANA – HALF BRIDGE POSE

This back stretch has a nice sensual feel, the upper back is lifted and the top of the pelvis well stretched out. The form of the stretch is similar to one which you might make standing up and having a langorous stretch in the morning, but because the body is supported on the floor the curves can be intensified and aligned.

Begin in *salamba sarvangasana*, the shoulder stand.

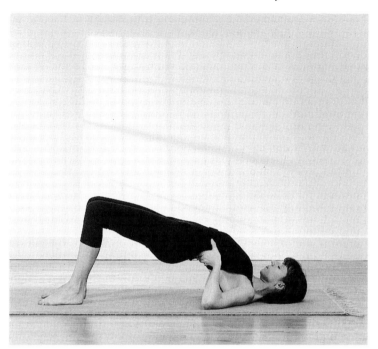

Setu bhandasana (half bridge pose)

Supporting your upper back with your hands, bring your elbows as close together as you can (ideally the upper arms on the floor should be parallel). When you are first learning to do *setu bhandasana* you may find it useful to arrive at the floor like this: keeping the lift up between your shoulder blades and your breathing steady, bend your right knee slightly and draw your right leg towards your chest. With a feeling in the left hip of arching up and over, take your left leg down towards the floor. When you feel stable, take your right foot up and over, down to the floor as well.

When the pose is familiar and you feel confident in it, you will find you can give a lift to your hips, and drop both feet lightly to the floor together. Try to land lightly like a cat.

When there is more extension there, walk your feet away until your legs are straight and bring your feet as close together as possible. Keep your tail bone lifted and enjoy the spreading feeling in the front of your pelvis.

If it feels extremely uncomfortable in your hands or your hips to do this pose, try bringing your feet down onto a low stool or a heap of cushions first (arrange them up against a wall or heavy piece of furniture so that they don't skid away when your feet come down), or use the wall itself: come up into the shoulder stand position close enough to be able gradually to walk your feet down the wall as your flexibility increases.

To come out of *setu bandhasana*, exhale, bending your knees, then unwind your hips, the back of your waist, your upper back, and then the lengthened back of your neck onto the floor. If the back of your waist feels tight, hug your knees to your chest, and rock gently from side to side.

OVERSTRESSED

Mental and emotional stress, along with physical stiffness, is one of the invisible epidemics of the last decades of the twentieth century. A certain amount of stress is, of course, challenging and stimulating, and can help us to develop and excel. Beyond a critical point – different for each individual – it becomes destructive. We perform tasks less well, make more errors and begin to suffer from physical manifestations of stress such as disturbances in sleep and digestion, panic attacks accompanied by perhaps palpitations, extra sweating, shallow fast breathing and so on. We are all familiar with these results of stress, and many of us have experienced some, if not all of them.

Yoga affects stress levels in many ways. Physically speaking, stretching, steady breathing, relaxation and meditation all help to disperse the stress-produced hormones, particularly adrenalin, and encourage the production of hormones which give a sense of well-being.

At a mental or spiritual level, a different perspective on life begins to arise over the weeks and months of practice. This does not imply that one will be any less committed to either career or family, but that there will be less sense of helpless entanglement. A growing sense of the value of inner experience, other people's as well as one's own, of the longer perspective of time and the wider issues of the world, tend to decrease day-to-day stress. This is very valuable to women who may find themselves extended by coordinating a career and children, perhaps also supporting and counselling a worried partner and having an increasing sense of responsibility for ageing parents.

If taking a broad view of the planet brings you another kind of stress, trying to work out what you can do to help preserve the ecosystem, look at Joanna Macey's book, *Despair and Personal Power in the Nuclear Age* (see Further Reading), which helps to find a way of living with the knowledge we have about pollution and arms.

When practising postures, *savasana*, breathing and meditation, the work involves being fully present in the present moment. This continual full attention to each successive second gives a relief from stress and a vivid experience of your own presence in the world. It is described by Dainin Katigiri thus:

> We do not realize it, but mind is always picking up activity right at the moment of activity. When you pick up activity, immediately it is form or experience. But right in the midst of activity, there is no form. All you have to do is just be there. This is oneness.
>
> Oneness is the rhythm of the sameness of ocean and you. At that time it is called 'to swim'.
>
> From *Returning to Silence: Zen Practice in Everyday Life*,
> Dainin Katagiri, Shambhala, 1988

'Just being there' is the freedom from stress inherent in the deepest yoga, being in our own place in the world as fluently as if we were swimming in the ocean. Take care not to let your yoga become another stressor, by getting anxious and guilty if you have not done 'enough'. Do not say to yourself, 'Ought I to do some yoga now?' but, 'Would I like some quiet time for myself? Would I like to spend some of that time on yoga?' Ask yourself, 'What is right for me for today?' and act on that.

The imagery, as well as the physical aspect, of these postures may appeal to you if you are under a lot of stress.

Integrate them into your balanced programme.

GARUDASANA – EAGLE POSE

Garudasana is the pose of the eagle. In it the eagle becomes extended and soaring in the sky, then comes down to settle onto its nest, folded and quiet. Performing the pose helps to remind us of moving from extroversion, pouring out of energy and activity to introspection, gathering in of energy, and arriving at a quiet centre.

Begin in *tadasana*. Lift up tall and keep your eyes, mouth and throat soft, your shoulders releasing back and down. Drop your tail bone and lift your abdomen lightly. Feel your limbs are strong and alive.

When you are ready, on a breath in, lift your arms out and up to the extended position shown in the drawing.

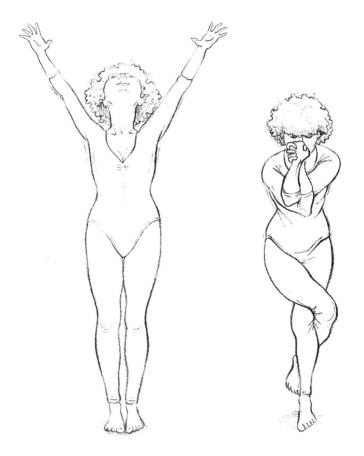

Garudasana (eagle pose) stage 1   *Garudasana* stage 2

Hold this position for a few steady breaths. Think of the huge, strong eagle, wheeling high above the plains. Feel the strength, the freedom, the sharpness of vision.

After a few breaths, allow yourself to feel your longing for quiet, for peace, for home. Breathing steadily, fold first your legs, then your arms, slowly into the twined eagle position. If your right leg is on top, let your left elbow be on top, and vice versa. Finally bend your standing leg a little more and incline your upper body forward, squeezing and warming your abdomen. Feel you are safely folded and curled onto your eyrie.

After a few more breaths, gently unwind yourself, and repeat *garudasana*, this time standing on the other leg, with the other arm on top.

You may need to practise this pose in two parts at first, becoming familiar with the leg and then the arm positions. If your legs will not wrap round each other twice, just cross them at the knee at first, and greater flexibility will gradually come into your ankles from practice of standing postures and work on lotus pose (*padmasana*), which will enable you to cross at the ankles too.

If your arms will not wrap round each other twice, cross them at the elbows and have the palms parallel, upright and facing outwards, until more stretch in the wrists enables you to cross at the wrists also.

Once you have become familiar with both the arm and leg positions, you can do them together in the balance. Keep your gaze resting steadily on one point and you will find it easier to balance. Even so, you may well, in the early stages of becoming familiar with *garudasana*, find yourself pogo-ing around the room in a most un-eagle-like manner. Do not worry. With practice, you will find you can manage the stretch and then the balance in a dignified way!

SUPTA BADDHA KONASANA – RECLINING COBBLER POSE

It is very relaxing to combine lying down in *savasana* with one of the hip-opening postures, like *baddha konasana* (cobbler pose).

Arrange yourself comfortably on the floor, lying on your back. Make sure you align yourself symmetrically around your spine. Check that the back of your neck is long – if there is tightness in your neck, roll it slowly and gently from side to side until it is eased, and then bring it back to the centre. Roll your arms away from your sides until your shoulders feel open and if you want to, shift your shoulder blades down a little towards your waist. Your hands are soft and curled like a little child's.

Bend your knees up, feet flat on the floor, and think of the lower back spreading and releasing. Push the soles of your feet together, and slowly let your knees fall out to the sides. Bring your heels in as close to your perineum as you can, and let your knees go down as far as possible. If you want to, shift and adjust your hips until you feel comfortable and symmetrical.

After a few breaths, you may want to stretch your arms straight up over your head to get an even fuller stretch, or stretch your arms up and then fold them onto the floor above your head, holding onto opposite elbows.

Feel very open and relaxed. Imagine you are floating in this position in a warm, blue lagoon. Imagine that the warm sun is soaking into your body and a gentle breeze flickering over your skin.

When you are ready to come out of the pose, bring your knees up and rest your feet flat onto the floor. Hug your knees up onto your chest and rock from side to side a few times, then roll over onto your side and push your hands into the floor to help yourself sit up.

HALASANA - PLOUGH POSE

The plough pose is a development from *salamba sarvangasana*, the shoulder stand (page 51).

After lifting and aligning in shoulder stand, think of continuing to lift between your shoulder blades, and lift your hips as high as you can. Slowly lower your straight legs down towards the floor behind your head. If your legs are not yet loose enough to reach the floor, begin again with a chair or low stool behind your head so your feet can rest there until more flexibility comes in the feet and hips.

Once in *halasana*, think of making plenty of space between your face and your knees, this will help to give a lifting feeling to the pose.

This is a quiet and restful pose which gives a lovely stretch all along the back of the body.

If you feel there is still some more stretch available in your hips and legs, move into *karnapidasana* (knee to ear pose) by dropping your knees down beside your ears. Gently press your knees into your ears. If you wish, thread your hands over your knees and press your palms over your ears.

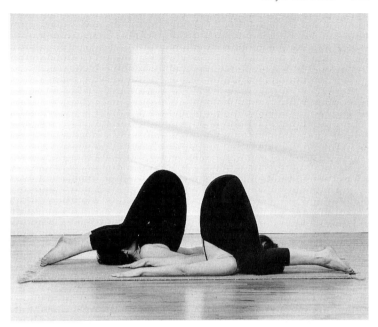

Halasana (plough pose) and *kamapidasana* (knee to ear pose)

To come out of *karnapidasana*, return to *halasana*. To come out of *halasana*, support your upper back with your hands. Unwind your back onto the floor a little at a time, drawing your legs along your face. When your back is on the floor, bend your legs and squeeze your legs onto your chest, rocking from side to side a little if you feel tension in your lower back. Think of your lower back spreading out. Place your feet flat onto the floor, then roll over onto your side before sitting yourself up.

UNDERSTRESSED

It can be as unpleasant to be understressed as it is to be overstressed. We are as likely as women to have parts of our lives when we do not have enough to do as we are to have stages when we are very hard pressed – for reasons of the fluctuating needs of our families, or of temporary bouts of unemployment due to house moves based on the requirements of partners' careers, or any of the other changes of location or focus that can happen. It is unpleasant to find your skills unused and your talents unchallenged, and not always easy to know where to begin to find an outlet for their expression.

SURYA NAMASKAR - SALUTE TO THE SUN

The series of postures known as *surya namaskar* or 'salute to the sun' is an enlivening and encouraging exercise.

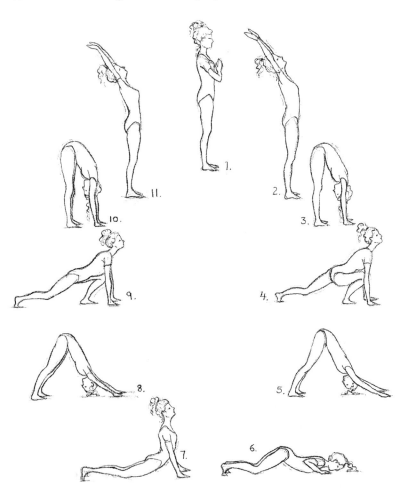

Surya namaskar (salute to the sun)

You will see from the illustration that it includes *tadasana*, the jack-knife (number 3), dog pose (numbers 5 and 8) and cobra pose (number 7) in an invigorating sequence. You can practise in a variety of ways: flowing from one position to the next slowly and remaining for a few seconds in each stretch, or swinging from one position to the next (avoiding any jerkiness or awkwardness) in a faster rhythm without pausing longer in each stage than it takes to fully extend in it.

Alternate the foot which you step back in position 2 each time you do the sequence. Do a couple of cycles on each side at first. You will find you feel energized and well stretched all over. When you have become more flexible and more fit, you can build up to several cycles on each side.

If you have little time for yoga, a few cycles of *surya namaskar* each day will help to keep you loose, active, and in touch with your body.

If you are feeling sluggish, bored and underused, the sequence will help to enliven you, and may help to loosen up your spirit too, enabling you to think of how to enrich your life and become more active and engaged in things which you enjoy and do well.

FEELING FRAGILE

Sometimes it seems to me that the reason women do so much crying is that they do a lot of other people's crying for them as well as their own. Women are often containing the emotions of other family members or friends who are unable to do this for themselves. In addition to this, frequently having to invent and re-invent a structure for an unstructured life, and cope with the physical impact of births, broken nights, crises and emergencies among colleagues, relatives and friends, can leave one feeling brittle and scoured out with strain and emotion.

The postures mentioned in the section on being alone will be helpful here because of their lifting and opening action on the chest and abdomen, and because they strengthen and revive the limbs, helping to stretch any feeling of wilting out of the body. The preliminary breathing exercises described at the end of Chapter 2 are also important. The use of breath to cleanse and refresh in this way can help to counteract the feeling, which is common when in a fragile state, that one can hardly breathe at all because each breath seems to hurt. Think of the breaths in flowing into you with a warm and nourishing kindness, and the breaths out taking some of the highly breakable feeling away with them.

VISUALIZATION IN *SAVASANA*

When you feel vulnerable and raw, combine *savasana* with a healing visualization. Read this several times over until it is clear in your mind and you can settle into *savasana* and let it flow in your imagination. You might otherwise prefer to put it onto tape and play it to yourself – if you have a tape-to-tape machine you can put some calm music following on from the visualization to let you continue to enjoy the feeling of peace and wholeness after it has finished. You may have a friend or partner who will read the visualization out to you when you have settled down. If you read onto tape or to a friend, read slowly, with pauses between the phrases as you feel appropriate.

Your body is heavy and relaxed . . . your joints are soft, your muscles warm and relaxed, your shoulders and hips feel heavy and open. Your head is heavy on the floor and your face is soft. Your hands and feet are soft and relaxed. Your spine is releasing more and more. Your breathing is coming and going lightly and steadily in its own rhythm. Your throat is passive and relaxed, and your mind is empty.

You are walking along a path towards a walled garden. There is a gate into the garden, and you are walking towards the gate. Go through the gate into the beautiful garden. The sun is deliciously warm on your body, and you soak up the warmth . . .

In the garden are beautiful flowers and shrubs all around you. Butterflies are dancing in the sunlight. You can smell the lovely scents arising from the warm flowers and you wander among the flower beds enjoying the colours, the shapes, the perfumes . . .

The sun is warm, it is peaceful, quiet and sleepy, just the occasional murmuring of bees or birdsong arises from time to time in the silence . . .

In the middle of the garden is a pool of clear, clean water.

You walk to the pool and dip yourself into the clear, clean sparkling water. All your tiredness, sadness and confusion is washed away in the crystal water of the pool.

Come out of the pool fresh and clean, newly born, and lay yourself down to dry in the warm sunshine, surrounded by the beauty of the garden . . .

Allow yourself as much time as you want and need to rest at the end of the visualization. When you are ready to bring your awareness back into the room and the situation you are in, do so by lengthening your breath a little, stretching first your fingers and toes, then your arms and legs, and having a good yawn, before you blink your eyes open and roll over onto your side, pushing your hands into the floor to sit yourself up.

If you enjoyed this guided fantasy, you will find more in Chapter 5.

VERY FIT

In contrast with the days or weeks when our consciousness of ourselves is of a breakable little shell, there are times too when we feel strong, magnificent, sturdy and marvellous. These strong poses are enjoyable to attempt while you are celebrating your strength. However exuberant you feel, do not forget all the usual cautions about not forcing, going in your own time to the rhythm of your own breathing, and not allowing pride or ego to cause you to rush. Having said that, with careful attention you can enjoy the resources of your capable and delightful body. Any time you are able to feel this positive awareness of your own body, or share the feeling with others, or help to awaken this feeling in them, you are helping to free women from the cruel tyranny of physical stereotypes, and reclaim the joy of the physical self, the miraculous organism made of the materials you have borrowed from the universe for the duration of this physical life.

VIRABHADRASANA III – WARRIOR POSE III
The third of the warrior cycle, this powerful balance is tough to do but very enjoyable. There are two routes into *Virabhadrasana III* – try both and see which gives you a better posture.

You can approach the pose from *tadasana*: after a few moments concentrating in *tadasana*, step your left foot back about a foot and rest it on its toes. Inhale and take your arms out to the sides, shoulder level and palms downwards. As you exhale, rotate the palms upwards and stretch your arms up, bringing your palms together above your head. Keep your shoulders relaxed, don't let them hunch into your ears.

Breathe in again, and as you exhale stretch your upper body forwards and down, parallel to the floor, simultaneously raising your left leg up parallel to the floor behind you. Don't forget to breathe.

Rest your gaze on one spot on the floor, it will help you to balance. Try to feel fully alive all along your body, and feel the standing leg is strong and sure, with a broad, full footprint.

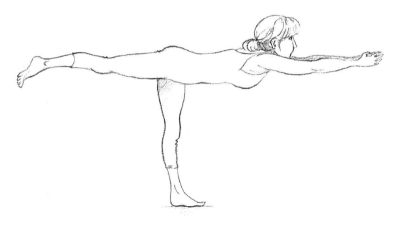

Virabhadrasana III (warrior pose)

Another way into *Virabhadrasana III* is to begin in *Virabhadrasana I* (see page 87). Inhale deeply, increasing your upward stretch, and then, as you exhale stretch your upper body forwards along your front thigh. As you feel your weight moving onto the front leg, press the foot into the ground and straighten the leg. Your back leg will naturally lift off the ground and as you come up you can adjust so that you are balanced with your back leg and upper body parallel to the ground.

The most difficult thing for most people is to turn the pelvis down so that it is open to the floor. It is tempting to roll the upper hip back. This is a time when you cannot see the pose, and it is difficult to reach back with your hand to feel what your hip is doing without falling over, so you may like to ask a friend or partner to observe your hips for you and tell you what is going on. If you want someone to adjust your hips, you really need two people to help, one to support your raised leg and help you to maintain your balance, and the other to adjust your hips very gently to a position where they are squarely facing the floor.

When you gain a firm balance in *virabhadrasana III*, remember the warrior. You could visualize yourself in a headlong charge, or the spear or arrow speeding through the air.

There are two ways to come out of *virabhadrasana III*. Either inhale and bring your body into an upright position, arms still extended overhead, and drop the back foot to the floor in a wide stride behind you. Then exhale, pivot your feet and turn your hips and shoulders to face forwards, stretch your arms out to the side, and lower them. Or, on a breath out, lower your hands to the floor near your standing foot and lower your raised leg to bring its foot down next to your standing foot. Come up from this forward bending position by inhaling and lifting your head, and exhaling, coming into an upright stance with your back broad and flat.

Do not forget to practise with equal concentration and for an equal length of time on the other side.

VASISTHASANA – INCLINED PLANE

Vasisthasana, the inclined plane, is a rather exciting development from dog pose, and can be made even more exciting by taking the top leg up with your fingers hooked around your big toe!

Begin in dog pose (*adho mukha svanasana*, pages 110–1). Exhaling, turn slowly to your left, opening your chest and hips to the left and laying your left arm along your side. Rest your left foot on top of the right and slowly ease your feet away from your supporting hand until the lower side of your body is in a straight line. Breathe steadily. As you breathe out, stretch your upper arm straight up in the air with your palm facing forwards. Look up at your upper thumb with your lower eye. Do not hold your entire weight up with the hand on the floor. Be aware of the activity in your hip and abdominal muscles, legs and shoulders, also working to keep you in the pose. Return to dog pose and, if you wish, drop

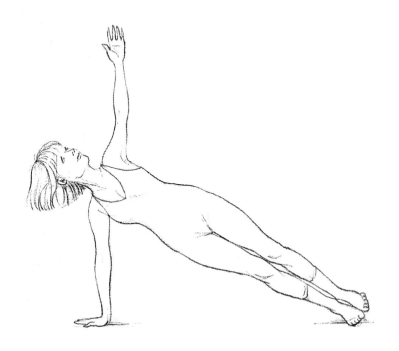

Vasisthasana (inclined plane)

down into the pose of the child for a few moments' rest before coming up into *vasisthasana* on the other side.

When you become familiar with this pose, try bending your upper knee and catching the toes of the upper foot, then exhaling and stretching the upper leg straight up. Look straight ahead and focus your gaze in order to assist yourself in the balance. Don't forget to work equally on the other side.

NATARAJASANA - LORD OF THE DANCE

Nataraja is one of the names for Siva, the Cosmic Dancer. The pose is beautiful, but harder than it looks, requiring great flexibility in hips, back, and shoulders.

Begin doing the pose by holding the bending leg with only the hand on the same side and with the elbow bending downwards rather than arching over the top.

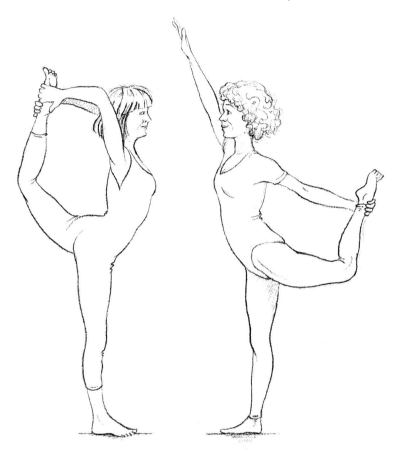

Natarajasana (lord of the dance)   Modified *natarajasana*

Begin in *tadasana* with a strong awareness of your contact with the ground and your long spine stretching forward. Steadying your gaze, bend your left knee and reach around behind with your left hand for your left foot. You may find it useful to hold your foot with the hand threaded round behind the instep rather than hooking over the top of it. Try both ways, and choose whichever is better for you. When you are ready, exhaling, stretch your right arm up into the air and push your left foot into your left hand, opening up the circle you see in the illustration. Only go to the right place for you for today.

When you are finished, exhale and release the posture, then do it again, balancing on the other leg. Make sure shoulder, hip and knee on the bending leg side are all aligned. It is easy to accidentally swing your knee out to the side in order to get a greater stretch, but this distorts the pose.

When you feel there is plenty of room in shoulders, hips and upper thighs, you can try the stronger version of the posture, with the bending leg lifted high and the elbows arching up and over. Some adepts are able to rest their head back onto the instep of the lifted foot! Never force the pace of this powerful stretch. The circle is the cycle of creation and destruction – the dance of life.

chapter five

IMAGE AND LIFESTYLE

Physical asanas are the route through which the majority of us in the West find our way to yoga. These asanas, however, are only part of yoga, so in this chapter we look at the guidance and interpretations we may find in yoga for a variety of different aspects of our lives.

EATING, SIZE AND WEIGHT

> Moderate diet means pleasant, sweet food, leaving free one fourth of the stomach.
>
> *Hatha Yoga Pradipika*, 1:58

Let's take the quality of the food and the quantity of the food as two separate issues. What, from the yoga point of view, is 'pleasant, sweet food'? Food, as well as all the other substances in the physical world, and as well as intangibles such as actions and motives, are divided into three different basic qualities known as the *gunas*: *sattva* (representing purity), *rajas* (representing activity, passion and the process of change) and *tamas* (representing darkness and inertia). These three qualities exist in the universe in a constantly shifting equilibrium, and are only transcended in a state of enlightenment.

The *sattvic* foods include cereals, wholemeal bread, fresh fruit, fresh vegetables, pure fruit juices, milk, butter, cheese, légumes, nuts, seeds and honey.

Rajasic foods include anything that is very hot, bitter, sour, dry or salty. Sharp spices and strong herbs are *rajasic*, as are coffee and tea, fish, eggs, salt and chocolate. It is considered *rajasic* to eat food in a hurry.

Tamasic foods include meat, alcohol, tobacco, onions, garlic, fermented foods, vinegar, and also anything which is stale or over-ripe. Overeating is *tamasic*.

The 'pleasant, sweet food' of the *Pradipika* refers to foods in the *sattvic* category, and we can aim gradually to eat more and more foods in the *sattvic* group, and less and less foods from the *rajasic* and *tamasic* types. Apply to any changes in your eating pattern the same attitude as you apply to your postures and your preliminary breathing exercises: that is, don't force anything, don't do anything that feels violent or awkward or extreme. Find that point of equilibrium in action where you are making choices not out of guilt, loyalty or dogma, but because those choices have arisen genuinely inside you. Eat a wide variety of foods within the *sattvic* category and, if you find you want less meat as you practise yoga more, be sure to have plenty of protein from other sources (nuts, pulses, cheese, and milk). *Sattvic* foods may look very bland at first and you may be alarmed at the thought of 'giving up' hot spices or coffee for example. However, it is probably better not to see it as an exercise in cutting things out of your intake, but rather noticing and allowing yourself to follow an increasing desire for fresh, rather plain food, and then enjoying the light, clean feeling that evolves from that.

Our planet is so polluted that it is very difficult to find foods free of excessive chemical toxins. It is, by now, probably impossible to find any food completely free of such substances which are spread throughout the soil, the air, the rain, and the oceans worldwide. We have to accept the fact that we can no longer clean up our food and our insides by taking individual responsibility for doing so, and understand with sorrow that it is already too late for that. What we can do is to wash all fresh fruits and vegetables thoroughly to rid them as much as possible of pesticides and lead, and use organically grown vegetables and grains where possible. We can be aware that both the antibiotics and the growth hormones fed to farm animals are present in most of the meat in the shops, and look out for organically raised meat if we want to eat meat. Fish absorb the waste poisons dissolved in the sea and rivers – the deeper swimming fish tend to be the cleanest, and fish such as eels and mussels which live in the shallows, the most polluted.

We can do our best to sort out our own food and eating, and to be informed and aware of news and research about pollution and its effects on ourselves and our families via the food we eat. The anger and sadness that we feel about this may prompt us to look for social as well as personal changes. In this everyone has to make her own choices about her own actions and her own boundaries.

The quantity of food to be eaten is clearly described: '. . . leaving free one fourth of the stomach.' Most animals eat what they need and no more. Half the human population of planet Earth cannot find enough to eat at the end of the Twentieth Century. Those of us in the fraction living in the affluent West often overeat. We have a very complicated relationship with quantity of food which leaves us in difficulty recognizing what it would feel like 'leaving free one fourth of the stomach', and even if we could sense what that was, we might find it difficult to stop eating there.

The rules, punishments and rewards concerning food which we experienced when we were children may have an effect on how we feel in our adult lives about the amount we eat. Women who were children in the UK when food was still rationed in the 1940s and early 1950s may have been aware of the adults' anxiety about food, whether there would be enough, and may have been very clearly instructed to eat everything they were given whether they felt hungry or not. Any woman who grew up with these pressures may feel obliged to 'eat up' leftovers, and always to finish everything on the plate. She may still carry a fear that there may not be enough food to last, so that nothing must ever be wasted, whether her body needs anything at that particular time or not. Although no-one would advocate wasting food, it may be useful to work on realizing that there is a choice, that food does not have to be finished up compulsively when it is not appropriate.

Women a decade or more younger may have been children when sweets finally came off ration in the early 1950s. Parents were delighted to be able to provide their children with sweets at last, and many of us had sweets every day for years through our childhood and, furthermore, the sweets were associated with rewards and pleasure, and withholding sweets was a form of punishment. Many of us thus linked in with refined sugars as a way of being nice to ourselves and other people, and came to associate a lack of sweets and chocolates with bleakness and punishment. Again, we may wish to re-examine that relationship with sweets so that we can choose when and how much to have of them with less of the emotional complications.

Still younger women may have had their relationship with food affected by the growth of the fast food industry, and become accustomed to large amounts of highly processed foods of all kinds. Social restrictions on having snacks between meals and on eating while moving around were relaxed and many people have become used to eating something as soon as they feel even a little bit hungry, rather than eating regular meals in-between which they expected to feel hungry at times. A change to more fresh wholefoods should be made gradually in order to let the digestive system accustom itself to fresh foodstuffs. Equally, a change to regular meals with spaces in-between rather than a continual stream of snacks should be negotiated gradually.

In spite of the fact that women in the Third World spend their entire lives trying to find enough to eat many of us in the West are pulled into the cultural obsession to be thin, and disrupt our eating patterns and our metabolisms by repeatedly going on and off more or less radical diets. The desperation to control our weight and size can sometimes become a metaphor for an attempt to control our lives and identities, and when that happens the acute suffering of anorexia nervosa and bulimia nervosa may become a possibility.

If you feel larger than is comfortable for you, you might want to consider gradually eating smaller quantities of fat, and moderate quantities of complex carbohydrates, filling up more with vegetables and fruits. Towards the end of a meal, think about leaving a fourth of your stomach free. Don't tense up about it, but think about how full or not you feel. Give yourself a few moments to make a choice about whether to go on eating or not. Notice the difference between how your abdomen feels when you have filled your stomach up completely, and when you leave it a little empty. Do what feels right for you at that particular moment, and also notice how you feel in the following few hours and whether your decision has affected that or not. We *can* gradually learn to eat only what we need, but it takes time and we need to be patient with ourselves.

Kim Chernin's book, *The Hungry Self* (see Further Reading) looks at women's struggles with a bulimic relationship with food and identity, and Sheila Macleod's *The Art of Starvation* (see Further Reading) tells her own story of episodes of anorexia. These books are useful to all women because they illuminate the way in which food and identity have become tangled for women. If you or anybody close to you is suffering from anorexia or bulimia you must understand that these are life-threatening conditions and seek help through your GP or by going straight to a centre specializing in eating disorders. Practising yoga is an excellent way to help to rebuild a loving relationship with the physical self, and to dismantle punitive and destructive feelings about the body, and is therefore useful to any woman suffering in this way.

To sum up, then, gradual change to a moderate, *sattvic* diet without making a fetish of it and learning to eat to about three-quarters fullness and to stop there, again without making a battle of will and self-discipline about it, should help to make our bodies arrive at the size and weight that is comfortable, healthy and appropriate for us as individuals.

Consider the *gunas* once again: *sattva* meaning purity, *rajas* meaning activity and passion and *tamas* meaning inertia and darkness. Once you have absorbed the idea of these categories you can see how they could apply to other substances, and also attitudes and forms of behaviour: for instance, you can imagine the differences between *rajasic* touch, *tamasic* touch and *sattvic* touch, differences which would be important in massage or even the most informal kind of healing touch. Consider making *sattvic* choices a greater part of your life in order to increase your feeling of well-being and inner quiet. It may seem unlikely that you could prioritize *sattvic* behaviour in, say, a business context or on a social occasion, but it does not actually involve being weak, passive or dull, rather a peaceful alertness and a liveliness that comes from inner aliveness instead of a brittle performance. Do not allow these considerations to make you become self-conscious and confused – simply carry the idea around with you and see how and where it might apply usefully for you.

CHAKRA, COLOUR AND SOUND

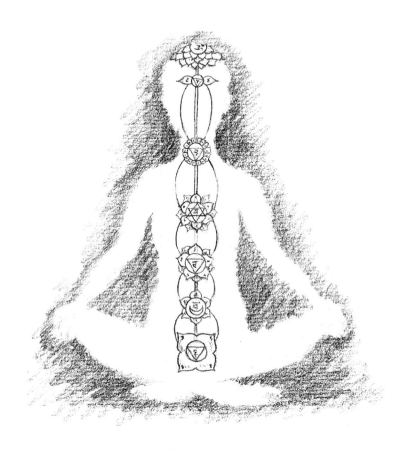

The *chakras*

The *chakras* are energy centres which lie along the centre line of the body. Each *chakra* relates to particular activities, moods and qualities, as well as colours and sounds.

Some practitioners of yoga regard the existence of the *chakras* as the literal truth, some would see them as symbolic or metaphorical. It is a matter for each person to work out for herself, and indeed one's views may change as one makes a stronger link with yoga. The location of the *chakras* corresponds with plexuses in the physical body, but this does not either prove or disprove that they 'really' exist.

We may also notice that there is a congruence between some of our own cultural locations for feelings in the body, such as putting our hand over our heart, which corresponds to *anahata chakra*, the *chakra* for emotional harmony, while describing strong emotions; or pressing the fingers into *ajna chakra*, between the eyebrows, which is the *chakra* for intellectual activity, when we are struggling to understand a complicated concept. This does not 'prove' or 'disprove' the existence of the *chakras* either, but it is an interesting resonance.

Perhaps the most useful approach is to begin by assuming that the *chakras* are an interesting set of symbols – like, for example, Jung's archetypes of the collective unconscious – and see what insight and growth proceeds from responding to them at that level. You can then see whether a further sense of the meaning of the *chakras* develops for you later on.

Colours in the Chakras

Each *chakra* has a corresponding colour. When you imagine the location of the *chakra*, imagine a glow of its colour in that place. You may also like to think of the colours which you enjoy wearing in terms of their *chakra* meaning, and sometimes to choose clothes, or even a small item such as a scarf or jewellery, of a colour to vibrate with the *chakra* energy you feel you need. We are all aware of the fact that our sense of confidence and well-being is influenced by the clothes we wear, and that something that 'feels' right and looks lovely one day may feel and look quite incongruous the next.

Muladhara chakra is situated at the perineum. Its colour is red, and wearing red or red objects helps to stabilize and earth a person. There are many different reds – look carefully – some sing with an undertone of yellow and orange, some with vibration of blue and violet. Some are a pure tulip red. If your red has undertones of other colours, it will carry a slight undercurrent of those *chakra* energies too.

The activities associated with *muladhara chakra* are action, sensation and reproduction, and the mental process is that of establishing facts.

Swadisthana chakra is located at the prostatic plexus and relates to the colour orange. Orange is a propitious colour for interaction and making changes, and helps with sociability. You may like to wear orange clothes or accessories if interaction with others is important for you at a particular time.

Activities associated with *swadisthana chakra* are social interaction; the mental process is that of relating and making comparisons.

Manipura chakra sits at the solar plexus and its colour is yellow. Wearing yellow helps to support the ego and self-confidence, and is an antidote to depression. Think of how your heart lifts when you see the first daffodils of spring! The colour is a wonderful celebration. Pale-skinned northern races hesitate to wear yellow, since the colour seems to drain tone from a white skin, but if you are white-skinned, look for a yellow with a golden undertone rather than with a blue or a lime undertone, and you will find it easy enough to wear.

Activities which relate to the *manipura chakra* are intellectual explanations and analysis.

Moving up the *sushumna*, the central channel of energy corresponding to the spinal cord in the physical body, the next *chakra* is *anahata* at roughly heart level. Its function is to harmonize at the emotional level, and its colour is green. Green is a pleasant colour to wear if you feel crowded, rushed or pressurized emotionally, but should be avoided if you are feeling over-emotional, as it will only activate your emotions even more. Be aware of the undertone colours in any green you choose.

Anahata-based activities are the search for security and self-esteem.

Vissudha chakra is in the throat and its colour is blue. The *vissudha* activities are study, learning, absorbing facts – not so much the intellectual-insight side of study which is the province of *ajna*, but more the hard work and application, highly verbal and logical side of study and learning. Perhaps scholastic organizations are inclined also to have particular songs linked with them to refresh *vissudha chakra* with singing after long hours of study! Blue is a good colour to aid concentration, receptivity, and learning.

The activities linked with *vissudha* are being in authority, learning about the past, and synthesizing data into concepts.

Ajna chakra sits in the third eye position between and slightly above the eyebrows. It is linked, as already mentioned, with intellectual insights, and with intuition and psychic qualities. Its colour is indigo.

The activities linked with it are direct perception and intuition.

Sahasraha chakra is the thousand-petalled lotus at the crown of the head. It radiates a pure and spiritual quality. The location of *sahasraha chakra* is the same as is highlighted by haloes in the religious paintings of Western art. The colours linked with *sahasraha* are white and violet. Many cultures use white garments to signify purity, especially on ceremonial occasions. White silk often has a delightful violet tinge, combining the two colours together.

The activities which arise from *sahasraha* are envisioning and the creation of images.

It would probably be a mistake to begin putting on clothes as it were 'for luck', linked with the *chakra* colours, in an artificial manner. It would leave you feeling self-conscious and silly. You might find it interesting, though, to think about the different colours you have chosen to wear in different parts of your life and notice whether they link in with the *chakras* in any way. I notice, for example, that when I first began yoga, long before I had heard anything about the *chakras*, I bought a red leotard. When this disintegrated a couple of years later I chose a green one, and on its demise a blue one was selected, still not having any idea what the colours might 'mean' in the *chakric* sense. Most of my life I have worn predominantly blue clothes and am indeed inclined to be rather bookish and very verbal.

In terms of choosing clothes, be intuitive about what you want to wear, rather than trying deliberately to pick the 'right' colour for the situation you anticipate. If you choose intuitively, you will often see in retrospect that you picked exactly the colour you needed.

The shape and texture of clothes can be thought of in terms of the *gunas*. As we discussed with relation to food, you will probably find that a desire to wear *sattvic* shapes and textures (natural fibres, fluid, highly physical, unrestrictive shapes) will evolve as you become more and more involved with your yoga practice. There is no need at all to begin changing artificially, as an affectation. It happens by itself in time.

Sound and the Chakras

The energy of colour affects us in one way and the energy of sound affects us in another way.

All of us have experienced both the location of different kinds of sounds from our own voices within our own bodies and also the profound effect on our emotional and spiritual state of hearing different sounds.

Think of how your voice rings in your own ears and vibrates in the skull area if you shriek or squeal. When you hum gently you may feel a warm buzzing feeling in the lips and a pleasant vibration in the rib cage. If you have experienced childbirth, you may recall extraordinary noises coming out of you quite involuntarily while you pushed the baby out – deep groaning sounds having a definitely pelvic origin. Sound can certainly be experienced in all sorts of ways and qualities throughout the body.

As for the emotional aspect, strong feelings can clearly be released by sound. Most of us find rhythmic sounds, the waves breaking on the beach, breezes rustling in the trees, very soothing. A sudden noise on a silent night can send a shudder up the spine. If a breeze grows to a hurricane, the sound of nature becoming violent makes the skin prickle, and the hair at the nape of the neck stir, while the pulse races. Gentle crooning or singing are soothing to hear from the earliest age, and if the song or tune is one we know, strong associative processes will bring back old emotions, sometimes very poignantly.

The sounds used in the yoga discipline are known as *mantras* (*man*: thinking; *tra*: a means of). Each *chakra* has its own *mantra*. While you repeat it you focus your awareness on the *chakra*.

When there is an 'a' sound in the middle of the *mantras* it is pronounced as a long 'ah'. The 'o' sound in the last two *mantras* is a long 'oh'. The *mantras* are as follows:

muladhara chakra	LAM
swadisthana chakra	VAM
manipura chakra	RAM
anahata chakra	YAM

vissudha chakra	HAM
ajna chakra	OM (shorter)
sahasraha chakra	OM (longer)

If you want to try chanting, begin by sitting with the spine lifting upright from its root to the skull and with your chest lifting and open, your shoulders releasing back and down. Relax your hips and knees in a cross-legged position or, if you are comfortable in either *siddhasana* or *padmasana* (the lotus pose), either of those would be suitable. Take your time getting established in a poised position, lifting but relaxed.

Let your eyes close and let your breathing steady itself into a rhythm. When your breathing is steady inhale, pause momentarily, then begin to chant. If you are chanting a *mantra* with three sounds in it, use about a third of the breath on each sound, and let the breath flow out at a steady pace. Choose any note you like, and experience the sound vibrating in your body. If you are using one of the *chakra mantras*, take your awareness to the site of the appropriate *chakra*.

When the breath is finished and the sound has died away, inhale at an even rate, without strain, and chant again. You will probably find five or six repetitions of the *mantra* will be enough at first.

It is refreshing to start at *muladhara chakra*, and chant the *mantra* for each *chakra* in turn, repeating each the same number of times, moving up the *sushumna*.

When you come to *ajna chakra*, the 'om' is chanted on a relatively high note and repeated several times with each breath rather like a bell chiming. *Sahasraha chakra* has a long 'om', where you think of the sound originating deep down in the hips and gradually flowing upwards to the crown of the head. It may be useful to feel the 'om' sound made of the flowing together of the sounds 'Ah-Oh-Mm'.

Approach chanting without strain or self-consciousness. The initial sense of oddness will soon fade. If you ever become dizzy, stop at once and let your breathing come to an everyday level until you are comfortable again. When you chant again, do not 'try' quite so hard. Think of pacing the breath out, with its sound, gently and evenly.

When you become used to chanting its initial effect is that mixture of soothing and energizing which is so characteristic of yoga practices. Later the repetition of *mantra* leads to a meditative state, stilling the current of thought and opening the door to an experience of oneness.

When you have become used to repeating a *mantra* out loud, you will find that it is also possible to concentrate on silent repetitions of the *mantra* and arrive at a similar state of peace and stillness.

YAMA AND *NIYAMA* – ON NOT GOING TO EXTREMES

Yoga gives guidelines on what might be called attitude or lifestyle. The *yamas* and *niyamas* are moral precepts which are prerequisites to the practice of yoga – in the eight-fold path (see Chapter 1) they come *before* posture (*asana*) and breathing/*prana* disciplines (*pranayama*). The frame of mind in which you undertake all your practice should be based on the *yamas* and *niyamas*. What precisely each *yama* and *niyama* means, and what its applications and limits are in your own life, is a matter for each person to work out, and frequently review in the light of experience.

Yama

The *yamas* are listed briefly on the following pages.

AHIMSA - NON-VIOLENCE
The concept of *ahimsa* needs careful thought. Does it for you include violence to humans? to animals? to the planet? Would offending somebody else's ideals count as violence for you? What if the other person was behaving in a way that you regard as over-sensitive? Where does your responsibility end and theirs begin? Would encroaching on the spirit of an occasion be violent in your view? These distinctions can only be arrived at with careful thought.

SATYA - TRUTHFULNESS
Clearly we all aim to be truthful over really important issues. However, is it all right to lie in order to oil the social wheels from time to time? Is it acceptable to lie to protect someone else? Is the literal truth more important than being true to the ideals of kindness and friendliness? Are there times when it is important to speak the truth even though it might hurt somebody else?

ASTEYA - NON-STEALING

Few of us steal other people's property. Is it equally important not to steal their time, or their credit, or their opportunities?

BRAHMACHARYA - CELIBACY

What does celibacy mean for us in our culture? Does it mean abstaining from sex altogether? Or does it mean abstaining from compulsive and exploitative sex? Perhaps the latter is more applicable, perhaps it is to do with looking at how you choose to spend your potential energy, and how you deal with very vivid sensations and experiences. Perhaps the concept of *brahmacharya* extends to other experiences where you might get drawn into a compulsive or exploitative reaction – the use of drugs or alcohol for example; or perhaps it applies to relationships other than sexual ones where the issues of possessiveness, faithfulness, and integrity could still arise.

Historically, some gurus have been literally celibate, while others have had partners and families. In paintings and drawings you will see some teachers sitting on tiger skins, and some on antelope skins. Only a complete celibate is permitted to sit on a tiger skin.

In the Eastern literature about yoga there is little reference to celibacy with regard to women. It is, however, a powerful theme in medieval Christian culture that a woman could increase her power, energy, and possible range of action in the world by becoming a member of a celibate order. She could also enter a contemplative celibate order and become an extremely powerful person and symbol in spiritual terms, and could claim special social status, respect, and rights as a result of her celibate state.

In the late Nineteenth and early Twentieth Centuries women had to make a clear choice between marriage and entry into professions such as teaching or the civil service. This is not to say that they were necessarily celibate if unmarried, but probably some of them were. The restriction on employment seems to suggest the residual feeling that a woman's finite amounts of potential energy had to be spent in properly chosen channels – either a family or a career but not both. Few of us would wish to return to any such restrictive practices and, indeed, seek instead to improve the balance between family and career by suggesting that male partners direct more energy into the home situation rather than women less into their careers. However, few women find the integration of multiple rôles simple. It may be what we want and have a right to, but it isn't easy.

Until the second half of the Twentieth Century celibacy was the only sure way for a woman to know that her work, efforts and development would not be punctuated by a regular stream of pregnancies, miscarriages and births.

Speaking in 1989, 18 years after the publication of *The Female Eunuch*, Germaine Greer reflected that, at present, women seemed to be liberated, only to be permanently exhausted; that they had successfully fought for the right for key jobs in the professions but had continued to do all their other types of work as well.

With these things in mind, the precept of *brahmacharya* may give a woman, as well as an opportunity to reflect on strategies and philosophies for avoiding compulsive and exploitative sex and sexuality, a chance to think carefully about the distribution of her energies generally, and whether they are being used in the ways which she would positively choose.

APARIGRAHA – NON-COVETOUSNESS

Aparigraha refers to not coveting objects belonging to someone else, as in the familiar Biblical commandment.

We need to consider whether it has any further meanings for us. Does it, for instance, extend to not coveting another person's talents and abilities, or physique, or career, or opportunities? Maybe it does.

Aparigraha further implies non-attachment to anything. Nothing, in the last analysis, really belongs to anybody. The body I live in, composed of and functioning by its use of gases, plants and animals that I consume and transform, can hardly be said to belong to me. It seems much more like something that I borrow, do my best or worst with, but ultimately have to give back to the universe after a number of years. Any abilities I have certainly do not belong to me – they evolve out of my circumstances and the way I choose to respond to those circumstances, but they can hardly be said to be property of mine.

Women have, very appropriately through the feminist movement, made efforts to reclaim their bodies from male definition, to name and celebrate their skills, strengths, and abilities. I have participated in this growth and been much strengthened and empowered by it – and practice of *aparigraha* need not undermine anybody's self-esteem – but it can suggest a perspective for assessing who owns what in the universe which may be useful.

As with the postures, the breathing, the rest of yoga, consider the *yamas* in whatever way and to whatever extent is useful for you for today. There is no need to come to definitive conclusions. They are like a crystal you might look at and see different refractions on different occasions – all of them real.

Niyama

Niyamas are not so much about the interactions between people as about one's frame of mind and way of living. It may be useful to reflect on these.

SAUCHA – PURITY

Saucha includes outer cleanliness like bathing and cleaning the body, and inner cleanliness effected by the practice of *pranayama*, and by *sattvic* eating.

Saucha also refers to a purity of the mind and spirit. Women have suffered so much from being the 'angel in the house', from being expected in this culture to be the 'nice' ones in any situation: pacific, diplomatic, flexible and generous, that this precept of mental *saucha* may be hard to contemplate. It does not, in my view, involve being passive, weak, or exploited. It implies rather a commitment and development towards positive and clear thought and action. It may militate against harbouring grudges, but it does not mean you have to give up righteous anger either on behalf of yourself as an individual, of women as a group, or of causes or issues about which you feel strongly. You do have an obligation to develop your thinking as lucidly as possible in order to make as clear a distinction as you can between unnecessary negative feelings and just anger, and to act positively to make such changes as you can when you feel your anger is just.

This is a personal interpretation of mine, showing clearly my reaction to an upbringing which conditioned me to be 'nice', hence my feeling of being very threatened by any instruction which seems to repeat that pressure to repress 'not nice' feelings or states of mind. No doubt some women will share that kind of conditioning and therefore arrive at a similar interpretation to mine. Others will have grown up in different contexts with different pressures and have different views. The important thing is to work out what the concept means for you in your particular life.

SANTOSA - CONTENTMENT

Santosa is contentment or tranquillity. Again, it does not mean helpless passivity, or pretending to like things which you do not like. It means, perhaps, a kind of acknowledgement of the reality of each minute as it comes along, such as is often described by the Zen teachers. A man who had a very tedious and demanding job asked Taknan, a Zen teacher, to suggest how he could get through the time. Taknan wrote eight Chinese characters and gave them to the man:

> Not   twice   this   day
> Inch   foot   time   gem

The interpretation is, 'This day will not come again. Each moment is a priceless gem.' (*Zen Flesh, Zen Bones*, Anecdote 32, see Further Reading).

I feel this does not mean that every day is lovely if only you look at it properly, but that every day is unique, and your unique self interacting with this unique day has its own unrepeatable and valuable flavour, whatever that may be. Reflection on this helps to dispel the discontent that arises when our days pass in a sort of grey soup, and a strange contentment, even in the presence of pain, pressure and other negative experiences can arise. At times it grows to a vivid pleasure about being in the world at all, whatever the conditions of one's life:

> There is nothing to see through our six senses. But when we sit down, we can exactly encounter what-is-just-is. Also within what-is-just-is, which is called buddha, we can become one with winter, trees, birds, all sentient beings, exactly.
> *Returning to Silence,* Dainin Katigiri, p. 55

Perhaps that feeling of belonging in, and identification with, the world, is where contentment can begin – or perhaps that is only where it begins for me. Ask yourself where it may begin for you.

Tapas – AUSTERITY

Tapas comes from the root word *tap* which means to burn, or blaze, or be radiant or brilliant. It may be thought of as the burning heat of effort and enthusiasm, or as a purifying fire which burns away the clutter of old anxieties, confusions and repressed emotions.

Most of us have an aspect which burns brightly – *tapas* acknowledges and celebrates this. It challenges us to consider whether we are burning in the place and in the way that we really would choose to burn: that is, are our best efforts and enthusiasms being used where we feel they really are best used.

Svadhyaya – STUDY

Sva means 'self', and *adhyaya* means study or education, so *svadhyaya* means 'education of the self' or 'study conducive to knowledge of the self'. Any activity which leads to exploration or enrichment of the self is practice of *svadhyaya*.

Ishvarapranidhana – SURRENDER TO Ishvara

Ishvara means the subtlest level of creation – the essence of creativity. *Ishvarapranidhana* means the dedication of all actions and thoughts, hopes and aspirations, to creativity, to growth and development, to positivity, energy and love. It implies a detachment from the short-term results and rewards for actions, and a commitment to act for the best without attachment.

YOGA NIDRA

Yoga Nidra is a form of meditation where the body is sleeping but the mind is awake. The aim is to experience a deep restfulness while at the same time being completely alert.

Lie down and arrange yourself on the floor in *savasana*, corpse pose. Make sure your centre line is straight, your shoulders and hips open and soft, and the back of your neck long. Feel how your head is heavy on the floor and your body is soft and heavy, your limbs relaxed and your toes and fingers soft.

First of all, observe your breathing. Do not interfere with the breathing at all, just observe it. Do not sleep. Your body is becoming softer, heavier, more relaxed, but your mind is calm and alert.

When your breath has settled into its own natural rhythm, begin to count your breaths. The breath in is one, the breath out is two, and so on. Count up to seven and then go back to the beginning, and count to seven again. Continue with this for a few minutes. Do not fall asleep. Observe gently as you become more deeply relaxed.

Now take your awareness to each part of the body in turn. Just observe the body, do not sleep. Begin with the toes on your left foot. Be aware of each toe in turn, then the foot, the ball of the foot, the top of the foot, the heel. Take your awareness to your calf, your knee, your thigh, your hip. Do not sleep.

Go to the right foot and be aware of each toe in turn. Think of the ball of the right foot, the top of the foot, the heel. Be aware of the calf, the knee, the thigh, the hip. Pause and observe each part. Take your time – but do not sleep.

Become aware of your abdomen, the left side of your waist, the right side of your waist, then the left side of your chest, the right side of your chest.

Take your awareness to your left shoulder, upper arm, elbow, forearm, and wrist. Be aware of your left palm, of each finger, and your thumb. Do the same on the right side – shoulder, upper arm, elbow, forearm, wrist, palm, and fingers and thumb.

Think of your neck and throat, your face, your head.

Now think of your whole body. Do not sleep. Let the time pass, floating by.

When you want to surface again, breathe a little more deeply, yawn and stretch. Open your eyes and become used to the light. Stretch and wriggle until you feel ready to roll over onto your side, and push your hands into the floor to sit yourself up.

Sometimes people experience the observing action of *yoga nidra* as a light or glow of warmth travelling around the body. Sometimes it seems like a lightly stroking hand. This form of relaxation is simple but very effective. Practised once or twice a week it will link you into a lake of calmness and strength which will be a great resource for you.

You may like to read and re-read the instructions until you are familiar with them, or ask a friend to read the instructions out slowly to you, with plenty of pauses, or put the instructions onto a tape. If you tape *yoga nidra*, you might like to add some peaceful music on the end, to accompany your complete relaxation, or you may just prefer to be in the silence.

VISUALIZATION

This guided fantasy can be used in a similar way to the one described in Chapter 4. Either familiarize yourself with it and then settle down and follow the visualization through for yourself, taking your time and allowing yourself to notice what arises for you, or ask a friend to read through the visualization, leaving plenty of long pauses, or another possibility is to make a tape of the visualization, perhaps adding some gentle music after the final words so that you can continue to lie and enjoy the peace.

Clear a space on the floor and switch off the telephone. Lie yourself down comfortably, with the centre line of your body straight, Roll your legs and arms outwards until you have a feeling of your shoulders and hips being open. If you want to, shift your shoulder blades down a little towards your hips. Sometimes it is useful to be aware of what your 'leading' shoulder is doing (right side if you are right handed, left side if you are left handed). If it feels contracted, soften it by imagining you are sending your breath there to warm and loosen it. Have the back of your neck long, your face soft, and your hand heavy. Your limbs are heavy and relaxed, your fingers and toes are soft. Your body is heavy and soft. Let your breathing settle to its own comfortable level. It will probably be light and soft.

Imagine that you are standing on a path which leads to the sea.

Notice what the path is like: is it broad and clear? Is it rough or smooth? Is it curved, or straight, or does it have many twists and bends? Are there gates, or obstructions? What is the landscape around you like? What is the weather like? Notice all the details of the scene which came spontaneously into your mind.

Walk along your path towards the sea. Be aware if it is easy or tiring, a short or a long journey. Look at the shore when you arrive at it and again notice the landscape, the weather and the atmosphere.

You are able to swim right down to the depths of the sea. Walk into the sea and swim deep down into the depths. Notice whether it is easy or difficult, notice how you feel, what you see, what the colours, shapes and sensations are.

Now it is time to come out of the sea. If you want to, you can bring something with you. Look around and see what you would like to bring. Take it with you, and come out of the sea.

You come out of the sea and onto the shore and find a path which leads to a mountain. What is this path like? Notice what the path is like and notice how you feel, Be aware of the sights and sounds, the weather and the atmosphere. Walk towards the mountain.

You climb to the top of the mountain. Is it easy or difficult? What is the surface of the mountain like to climb on? Notice what you feel like and what you can see and hear.

You arrive at the top of the mountain and sit down for a while. Look around you. Consider how you feel and what you are experiencing. Take your time and observe what is going on for you.

Now it is time to come down from the mountain. If you want to you can bring something with you. Look around and see whether there is anything you would like to take with you. If there is, take it. Come down the mountain again and onto the ground. Perhaps you have something with you from the depths of the sea, and perhaps you have something with you from the top of the mountain.

You are coming along a path which leads you back to your everyday life. How does this feel? Walk back towards your everyday life noticing what you feel, hear and see . . .

Now it is time to bring your awareness back into the room, and to finish your relaxation. Begin to breathe a little more deeply, until you yawn, then yawn a few times. Stretch first your fingers and toes, then your arms and legs, and blink your eyes open to become used to the light. When you are ready, roll over onto your side, push your hands into the floor and sit yourself up.

Have a few moments to collect your thoughts before you return to the activities of your day.

Allow yourself to reflect on the sights, sensations and sounds of your journey and on any objects you 'brought back' with you. Do not search for their 'meaning', but allow any meanings or messages they have for you to evolve in your mind in the days and weeks that follow.

chapter six

OTHER OPPORTUNITIES
AND EXPLORATIONS

This final chapter introduces a few more possible avenues of exploration.

EYE EXERCISES

It is beneficial to exercise the muscles which move your eyes just as it is to exercise any other muscles. Moving and toning up your eye muscles helps to prevent tension building up around your eyes and the clenched feeling that can grow around the temples and over the cheekbones.

It is no accident that our eyes are called 'the windows of the soul'. When your eye muscles are strong and able to relax, you may find your eyes are more expressive. You won't see that of course unless you spend a great deal of time looking in the mirror, but you may see the result of it in that you will be more able to communicate clearly and genuinely with others.

SIMPLE EYE EXERCISE

Sit comfortably with your legs crossed, or in *siddhasana* or *padmasana* if those positions are really comfortable for you. Make sure you are sitting on the centre of the pelvic floor and your spine is lifting, shoulders relaxed and brow and jaw soft. Breathe steadily and keep your head still when you move your eyes. Slowly look upwards as far as you can without moving your head, then smoothly and slowly move your eyes to look down as far as possible. Move your gaze up and down five times.

Now move your gaze to the far left, then smoothly and slowly across to the far right. Move your eyes to the left and then to the right five times, breathing steadily and keeping your head still. Be aware of your spine lifting, your abdomen being active, your hips open and your shoulders soft.

Take your gaze to the uppermost point and then move it round in a large circle in a clockwise direction. Repeat another four times. Next, sweep your gaze round in five circles anticlockwise.

Settle your gaze back to the centre.

Finish this sequence by holding up your index finger about a foot in front of your face. Focus your gaze on your finger, then on something significantly further away – the far wall if you are indoors, a tree or plant or whatever if you are out of doors. Move your gaze from your near finger to the far object and back again five times. Then again soften your eyes to an everyday relaxed position.

Rub your hands together to make them warm, then cover your closed eyes with your warm hands. Feel the warmth and softness flowing between hands and face. Your eyes are soothed by 'palming' like this. When you want to move on, separate your fingers and blink your eyes open behind your hands so that your eyes can slowly become accustomed to the light. When your eyes are used to the light, slowly float your hands down into your lap. These simple eye exercises can be included at the beginning of your yoga practice after centring, or at the end before *savasana*, or you can spend a quiet five minutes doing them as a calming and relaxing interlude during a hectic and stressful day.

TRATAK

The practice of *tratak* involves a cycle of gazing steadily at an object and then closing your eyes and holding the image of the object in your mind's eye. The effect is to steady the mind and gradually to still the kaleidoscope of mental activity.

You could use a candle flame as an object for *tratak*, or a flower, a crystal, or a shell or stone which you like. If you use a candle flame, practise indoors away from draughts which will disturb the flame. Some objects can be used equally well in or out or doors.

Practise *tratak* sitting down and arrange the object you would like to use about three feet away at eye level. Sit comfortably, cross-legged, or in *siddhasana or padmasana* if those are easy for you. Lift your spine and lengthen the back of your neck, soften and open your shoulders and hips, and let the abdomen lift lightly. Breathe steadily and keep your face and throat soft.

Gaze at the flame, flower, crystal, or whatever, Slow down the rate of blinking as much as possible, though if your eyes water, allow yourself to blink. Do not become tense through trying to avoid blinking. With your body upright and poised, your breathing steady and easy, become absorbed in what you see. Distractions will arise and peripheral thoughts will irritate you at first. Simply observe them and then draw your mind back to what you are doing.

After a minute or so, close your eyes and visualize your chosen object at either *ajna chakra* (between your eyebrows and slightly upwards) or *anahata chakra* (around the heart area). Quietly bring the image alive at the *chakra* you choose. After a minute or so again, open your eyes once more and gaze again. Repeat this cycle until you are ready to stop.

If you are using a candle carefully blow it out. You may like to dedicate the light as you blow it out to any person or issue that comes into your mind, or to reflect on the sentence, 'You are the light of the world.'

Rest for a little while in *savasana* before you return to the activities of your day.

HAND EXERCISES

Your feet will become more supple, sensitive and expressive, and you will experience them much more fully, through your practice of yoga. It is a good idea to give some time and attention to your hands, too. There are minor *chakras* on both the feet and the hands. That is why when you see someone doing, for instance, *trikonasana* (triangle pose) with full energy, the palm of the upper hand, facing forwards, is radiant. In *chakric* terms, that is why you might want to squeeze or hold someone's hand when you are in pain or feeling fear: it helps to activate your own energies for dealing with that pain or fear.

Our hands are poignantly human. When we see a new baby we are entranced by the tiny hands. Holding hands is a particularly intimate kind of contact. With our hands we have a thousand skills and abilities.

SIMPLE HAND EXERCISES

With your right hand, bend each finger of the left hand back as far as it will comfortably go. When you come to the thumb, bend it first backwards, then downwards along the inside of your forearm as far as it will go. Change hands and bend the fingers and thumb of your right hand with your left.

Now once again work on your left hand with your right. Starting with the little finger, take each finger in turn and circle it gently in its socket, a few times in one direction, an equal number of times the other way. Do the thumb as well. Change over and circle the right hand fingers in their sockets with the left.

Finish by shaking your hands briskly, from side to side, then up and down.

MASSAGE

Hand massage is delightful to give and to receive. You can do it with or without the addition of a lightly perfumed oil.

If you are giving a massage of any kind, collect your thoughts first so that you do not pass any of your own tensions on to your partner through your hands. Steady your breathing and think of peace and tranquillity flowing through your hands.

Take your partner's hand in yours and 'open' the palm by stroking from its centre outwards with your thumbs. Be aware of what you are feeling – tendons, bones, blood vessels, special strengths and individual shapes. When the hand feels open, support it in one of yours while you massage each finger and the thumb by squeezing and stroking each section of each digit in turn. Follow your instinct, explore the hand as it comes to you intuitively to do. To finish, support your partner's hand palm downwards in your own and stroke with long slow strokes the back of the hand, from wrist to finger tips. Gently release your contact with that hand and massage your partner's other hand, giving it equal care and attention. Be aware of any differences between the two hands.

When you have massaged both your partner's hands, change rôles and enjoy the experience of her or him massaging your hands.

Sometimes it is interesting for the person having the massage to talk about their hands while the massage is happening: what skills their hands have; any injuries they have suffered; any special feelings they have about their size, shape, texture and qualities.

MUDRA

Mudra means a seal, or a sealing posture. There are many whole-body postures in the discipline of yoga which are *mudra* postures, forming sealed circuits of energy – for instance, *baddha konasana* (page 47).

Circles formed by the thumb and each of the fingers are also *mudras*, each having a significance. You can either use these as a symbolic or metaphorical aid to your own concentration and reflection, or as a literal set of meanings, according to what feels right for you.

The *mudra* most commonly seen is a circle formed by the thumb and index finger, with the other fingers outstretched. It is known as *jnana mudra* or the 'gesture of the initiate'. The top joint of the index finger is tucked into the top joint of the thumb in *jnana mudra*. The index finger represents the individual soul, and the thumb the universal soul. The joining of the two represents knowledge and integration. Linking the thumb with the middle finger means linking with discipline; with the fourth finger means linking with vitality, and with the fifth finger, linking with intellect.

You can form your hands into one of these circuits when you are doing centring, or meditation, or *tratak* if it feels appropriate to you to do so. *Jnana mudra* is the hand *mudra* usually preferred for *pranayama*. You can also quietly join your fingers into any of the *mudras* that feel appropriate to you at any time. If making the hand *mudras* feels awkward or unnatural to you there is no need to do them at all unless or until you want to. If you need to settle your hands for meditation, *tratak* or breathing work and *pranayama*, rest them palm upwards, one inside the other in your lap, instead.

MORE WORK WITH BREATHING

Always work carefully and steadily with breathing awareness and breathing work. Do not strain or do anything that feels uncomfortable or stressful.

ALTERNATE NOSTRIL BREATHING

This breathing pattern will steady and deepen your rhythm. It is very calming and can be used to defuse panic. It is also a good cure for insomnia. Sit with your spine lifting and the back of your neck long. Your shoulders are relaxed and your hips open – your legs arranged either cross-legged or in *siddhasana* or *padmasana* (lotus pose). Your abdomen is active and lifting.

Rest the back of your left hand on your left knee and join the thumb and index finger. Rest the middle finger of your right hand between your eyebrows and up slightly. Check that you can close your right nostril with your thumb, and your left nostril with your fourth finger. As you become more accustomed to alternate nostril breathing, experiment with closing the nostrils with the minimum possible pressure.

Inhale through both nostrils, then close your right nostril with your thumb, and exhale through the left.

Inhale through the left. Close the left nostril with the fourth finger.

Release the right nostril, and exhale through it. Inhale through the right. This is a complete cycle.

Continue with this cycle, allowing your breaths to spread out. Be aware of how you are feeling, do not force or strain your breath in any way, and keep your body upright and poised. When you are ready to stop, continue until your next exhalation on the left, then take your hand gently away from your face and rest it on your right knee. Let your breathing return to an everyday level, and become aware of the room and your surroundings before blinking your eyes open to let in the light.

BRAHAMARI

To practise *brahamari*, sit upright with the hips open as in all the other breathing work. Rest the backs of your hands on your knees and join thumbs and index fingers in *juana mudra*. Inhale, partly closing the back of the throat, so that there is a slight snoring sound in the back of the throat. Exhale slowly, humming with a slight vibration, like a bee. The sound really vibrates in your head and throat, and the out-breath becomes long and complete. Do not force or tense up your neck, shoulders, or arms. Repeat *brahamari* between five and ten times. It is very refreshing if you feel congested in the head, and also helps to deepen your normal breathing if you are finding yourself in a cycle of shallow breathing.

SITKARI

Sit as for *brahamari*. To do *sitkari*, protrude your tongue a little between your lips. Inhale slowly through your mouth – this will make a hissing sound. Hold the breath for two or three seconds, then exhale slowly through the nose. *Sitkari* is a cooling breath, useful if you are feeling literally, or metaphorically, hot and bothered. It is said to improve the countenance: '... by repeating this (*sitkari*) the yogi becomes as beautiful as a god.' (*Hatha-Yoga-Pradipika* 2:54). However, it is not a conventional 'beauty treatment', rather a part of a whole philosophy which may make one more beautiful by being more in touch with 'the goddess' within.

YANTRA AND MANDALA

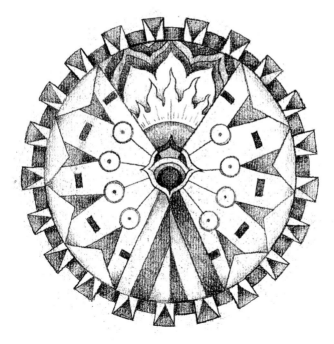

Yantra

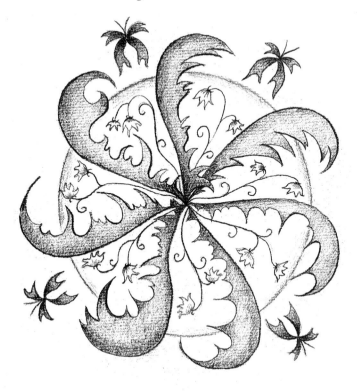

Mandala

Yantra and *mandala* are patterns which may be used for *tratak* or for continuous gazing and meditation. *Yantra* are usually geometrical in nature and tend to lead the eye in towards their centre, i.e. they are centripetal. *Mandala* may have a geometrical or a more fluid or organic look, and may contain representational pictures as well as pattern. They tend to lead the awareness to flow out from the centre and so their energy is centrifugal.

An upward pointing triangle in a *yantra* represents masculine energy, and a downward pointing triangle, feminine energy. They may sometimes be arranged on top of each other to make a star which represents harmony. A dot in the centre symbolizes the seed, the microcosm of potential. Circles in a *yantra* symbolize continuity – no beginning, no end, no dominance. Rectangular figures symbolize stability: the horizontal lines signifying repose, and the vertical lines signifying support. There may sometimes be stylized lotus petals included in a *yantra*, and sometimes a stylized rendering of the symbol for '*Om*'. The stillness of a *yantra* helps to settle and focus the mind.

Many natural organic structures are centrifugal like a *mandala*. Many flowers swirl or spread outwards like a *mandala* the way cells are packed in a plant stem, as you would see them sectioned through a microscope, is a *mandala*. The whorl of shells and shell fossils, the radiant effulgence around the sun setting among clouds, the earth itself, seen in all its innocent completeness from outer space by spacecraft, is a *mandala*.

The outward movement of energy in a *mandala* suggests a passage between different states – these can refer to general and cultural processes as well as private and inner ones. Movement, development and change, whatever those things represent to you at this particular moment, are elucidated by reflection on a *mandala*.

RAJA YOGA

Raja yoga is the name for the eight-fold path of yoga described by Patanjali in the yoga *Sutras* (see page 15). Much of the work suggested in this book is an interpretation of *Hatha* (posture) yoga and an approach to some of the other eight limbs: *pranayama* (work with breath and *prana*), *dharana* and *dhyana* (concentration and meditation). There are various other perspectives on a yogic life.

KARMA YOGA

Karma yoga is the yoga of action. It involves being clearly aware that every action in the world causes thousands of reactions and further actions radiating out from that initial action, and that we should therefore take deliberate responsibility for every action we make, however apparently trivial, because its consequences spread outwards to the very edges of existence.

Karma yoga also involves making a decision to act as well as possible, regardless of rewards or results: to do things fairly, or kindly, or well, for their own sake rather than for the expected outcome. This, therefore, is another example of detachment – detachment from results.

JNANA YOGA

This is the yoga of knowledge and wisdom, practised through study, reflection and meditation. When Westerners first come across yoga, they sometimes feel that they will be required to suspend their intellects in order to understand and practise it. This is not the case at all, and *jnana* yoga in particular requires the intellect to be extended and refined as much as possible in order to comprehend the interaction of all life and form within the universe, the working of the human body, the human mind, and social and economic structures in the world. Intelligent seeking of and use of information, and intelligent interpretation of information is *jnana* yoga, as is the exercise of the intellect in conjunction with all intuitive and imaginative activity.

BHAKTI YOGA

Bhakti yoga is the yoga of devotion and love. Careers and life-paths chosen for love, work done and efforts made for the sake of love for fellow human beings, fellow creatures, the planet itself, or a spiritual ideal, are all behaviour on the path of *bhakti* yoga. As far as yoga is concerned, any genuine act of love or compassion is an act of worship – in the same way as Christ expresses: 'inasmuch as you did this for the least of these my brethren, you did it for me' (*Matthew* 23:40).

Jnana, *bhakti,* and *karma* yoga are described in the *Bhagavad Gita*.

TANTRIC YOGA

Tantric yoga arose in India in about the fourth Century AD.

The use of *mantra*, *mandala*, *yantra* and *tratak* can be considered part of *tantric* yoga, where the practitioner uses physical experiences to induce or enhance mystical experiences. *Tantric* touch (frequently referred to in Ina May Gaskin's book *Spiritual Midwifery*) implies a touch fully aware of the spiritual connection between the toucher and the touched, and the spiritual channels between all of us and whatever kind of wider spiritual being or energy we believe in. Part of our growing awareness when we practise yoga is to do with learning not to touch people in an invasive or intrusive way, and in fact to make every touch a loving, or a gentle, or a healing touch. In some areas of life – in our loving relationships for instance – this may be relatively easy. In other areas – the underground train in the rush hour for example – it is more difficult! It should, however, be attempted.

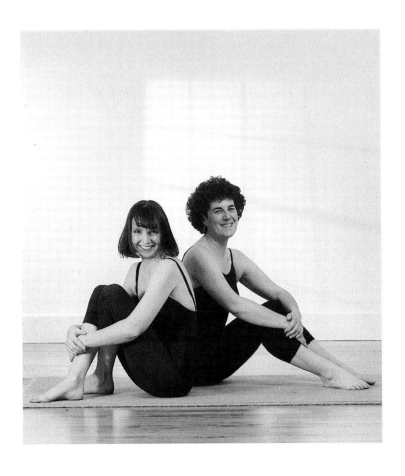

CONCLUSION

In this book we have looked at yoga, at what it might begin to mean and what it might offer to women beginning to consider it as we move towards the Twenty-first Century.

We have looked at postures which may build and lubricate and liberate the body, and the beginning of work with the breath and with stilling the mind which may begin to clear the mind of anxiety and bring a growing sense of peace.

We have also looked at awareness and revision of attitudes, and different perspectives on life. There is enough in the practices, the texts and the ideas of yoga to explore for several lifetimes.

It is everybody's individual choice as to how far you take your own search and research. In your journey you may like finally to bear in mind verse 13 from the *Yoga Sutras*:

The practice of yoga is the commitment
to become established in the state of freedom.

FURTHER READING

Effortless Being: The Yoga Sutras of Patanjali, trans. Alistair Shearer, Mandala, 1989

The Upanishads, trans. Shearer and Russell, Mandala, 1989

The Yoga of Light: Hatha-Yoga-Pradipika, trans. and commentary Hans-Ulrich Reiker, Unwin Hyman, 1989

Chakras: Energy Centres of Transformation, Harish Sohari, Destiny Books, 1987

Tao Te Ching (Lao Tzu), trans. Feng and English, Wildwood House, 1986

The Bhagavad Gita, trans. Easwaran, Arkana, 1985

The Dhammapada, trans. Easwaran, Arkana, 1987

Meditations with the Navajo: Navajo Stories of the Earth, Gerald Hausmann, Bear & Co, 1988

Returning to Silence: Zen Practice in Everyday Life, Dainin Katagiri, Shambhala, 1988

Stretch and Relax, Maxine Tobias and Mary Stewart, Dorling Kindersley, 1985

The Book of Yoga, Sivananda Yoga Group, Ebury Press, 1983

Double Yoga, White and Forrest, Penguin, 1981

Pranayama: The Yoga of Breathing, André van Lysbeth, Unwin Hyman, 1979

The Complete Book of Massage, Claire Maxwell-Hudson, Dorling Kindersley, 1988

The Body Has Its Reasons, Thérèse Bertherat, Cedar, 1976

Despair and Personal Power in the Nuclear Age, Joanna Macey, New Society Publishers, USA, 1984

Zen Flesh, Zen Bones: A Collection of Zen and Pre-Zen Writings, ed. Paul Reps, Penguin, 1971

The Hungry Self, Kim Chernin, Virago, 1986

The Art of Starvation: An Adolescent Observed, Sheila Macleod, Virago, 1981

INDEX